T0213842

Pioneers in Plastic Surgery

David Tolhurst

Pioneers in Plastic Surgery

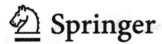 Springer

David Tolhurst
Department of Plastic Surgery
University Hospital Leiden
Leiden
The Netherlands

ISBN 978-3-319-36854-2   ISBN 978-3-319-19539-1   (eBook)
DOI 10.1007/978-3-319-19539-1

Springer Cham Heidelberg New York Dordrecht London
© Springer International Publishing Switzerland 2015
Softcover reprint of the hardcover 1st edition 2015

Printed on acid-free paper

Springer International Publishing AG Switzerland is part of Springer Science+Business Media
(www.springer.com)

For Camilla and Charlotte

Acknowledgements

The concept of this book was conceived many years ago when Barend Haeseker was one of my assistants during his training in plastic surgery. He is perhaps the world's leading historian and a prolific writer in Dutch on the subject of plastic surgery, and it is to his enthusiasm, knowledge and help with this collection of vignettes that I am greatly indebted.

I am very grateful to Penelope Hopwood for typing and retyping the text as well as crossing swords with me on the grammar and punctuation.

Finally my thanks are also due to family members of various pioneers, the librarians and archivists at the Royal College of Surgeons of England, the Wellcome Collection and the Sanvenero-Rosselli Foundation for permission to use photos and illustrations that are not in the public domain.

Contents

Introduction

There are two main reasons why we embarked upon the writing of this volume.

Firstly it is because history is a fascinating subject that interests not only the authors but also others in many walks of life. The stories surrounding the lives of well-known figures help to bring them back to life in the minds of readers. One other thing should not be forgotten, that is, the way in which history sets trends and thus puts the practice of modern surgery, for example, in its proper perspective. It gives the lie to so many sensational reports of miraculous new discoveries, which help to sell newspapers and magazines, that are often rediscoveries or blatant plagiarism.

To say that there is nothing new under the sun is an aphorism that takes the matter a little too far. However, diligent searching amongst the oeuvres of our forefathers nearly always reveals that someone, somewhere had put a finger on the subject in one way or another. For example, quite recently a reporter speaking on a BBC programme clearly stated that McIndoe was the founder of modern cosmetic surgery which is utter nonsense. He may have helped to increase its popularity, but others before he was born were already making important contributions to cosmetic surgery.

Secondly before one gets too carried away on history, we have put these vignettes together so that those who wish to glance into the past may do so and be spared the drudgery of searching through faded and dusty journals, half forgotten in some dreary, ill-lit corner of a library on a winter's afternoon. No doubt this book will come to rest in such a place, but before it does there is hope it will have reminded medical men and their patients alike that unless something is written on the work and lives of those who played a part in the founding of plastic surgery, their names and contributions will pass almost forgotten into oblivion. Much of the information on the stories of our chosen pioneers has been gleaned from obituaries and articles written by colleagues, and we are most grateful for their writings. The name plastische chirurgie appears to have been coined by Eduard Zeis, an ophthalmologist, in a publication in 1838. It was readily accepted on the continent as evidenced by its use in works written by French and German authors. Strangely there was nothing published in the English language during the nineteenth century under the title of plastic surgery although some of the most enlightened general surgeons exercised the principles of this discipline as part of their practice. Even though this type of surgery had been given a name, no one had decided to limit his practice to it alone nor had anyone announced or written that they were plastic surgeons until in 1909 when John Staige Davis of Baltimore did just that. It is for this reason that I have called him the 'first real plastic surgeon'. This did not mean that he was in any way superior to his colleagues as a surgeon for even in the nineteenth century, general or ENT surgeons such as Dieffenbach were perfectly competent and able to achieve fine results as is also the case today. In fact a number of procedures originated or perfected by plastic surgeons have now been 'claimed' by other specialties. For example, gynaecologists have maintained that breast surgery and vaginal agenesis should be surrendered to them. Likewise craniofacial surgery and even cleft lip and palate correction are now more frequently being undertaken by maxillofacial surgeons.

The word plastic has nothing to do with the material which is in universal use today. It was used to indicate the moulding or plasticity of the body's tissues. There has been some confusion over the term cosmetic surgery which some people mistake for plastic surgery. Cosmetic or aesthetic surgery has now been included in most responsible training programmes and from the early twentieth century has been accepted as part of the specialty of plastic surgery. Even in the British National Health service, it has been necessary for trainees to assist and carry out cosmetic operations, albeit in limited numbers. Some narrow-minded critics contend this is unacceptable. How then are young surgeons to learn the techniques? To some extent this explains why some surgeons such as Joseph, who devoted a lot of time to cosmetic surgery, have been chosen as early and influential pioneers in plastic surgery. To avoid confusion it is better to use a rather long-winded term such as reconstructive and cosmetic or aesthetic surgery rather than plastic surgery as a title. What was once the British Association of Plastic Surgeons is now lumbered with the title of the British Association of Plastic Reconstructive and Aesthetic Surgeons. For those struggling in the minefield of semantics, the Oxford Dictionary defines the word cosmetic as something 'designed to beautify the hair, skin or complexion', whilst aesthetic relates to the appreciation of beauty and taste.

In recent years there has been an enormous increase in the demand for cosmetic or aesthetic surgery, and such is the law in this country that any medical practitioner can call himself a cosmetic surgeon without the necessary training. Surgeons from other specialties and even general practitioners have watched or assisted at a few operations and then carried them out, realising there is a lot of money to be made in this way. Unfortunately unsatisfactory results and complications arising from poor surgery are more likely to develop in these situations. In some cases unhappy patients are then referred to plastic surgeons who may not wish to become involved with a difficult patient or are reluctant to do so because of the threat of litigation with the result that the patient may be left helpless. Recently steps have been taken to rectify this state of affairs with the organisation of proper training and certification of those wishing to practise cosmetic surgery.

The specialty of plastic surgery was accepted by Charles University in Prague in 1929, enabling Burian to appoint and train surgeons in his department. Three years later it was legally recognised in Czechoslovakia which appears to be the first country in the world to do so. Although the American Society of Plastic Surgeons was established in 1931, it was not until 1937 that a Plastic Surgery Board finally held its first meeting, largely due to the work of Vilray Blair, who agreed to act as secretary.

Much has been written on the development of the specialty, and there has even been confusion over dates and names of the pioneers, some of which we have attempted to clarify. The pioneers we have chosen were originally surgeons practising general, ear nose and throat or orthopaedic surgery who became interested in reconstructive or corrective operations and as a result spent much more or most of their time on plastic surgical procedures. Some names well known to today's surgeons have not been included as they will have only become relatively famous because of one idea or invention. Examples are Thiesch and Wolfe who put skin grafting on the map! That is not to say these people have not played an important part in the development of plastic surgery but rather a somewhat limited one.

Many of the pioneers were fascinating and sometimes multitalented people. Where possible we have endeavoured to describe these aspects of their lives more fully rather than concentrating on descriptions of surgical procedures so that readers outside the medical world may find not only the accounts of their work but also their adventures, personalities and peculiarities entertaining.

Chapter 1
Pre-nineteenth-Century Surgery

Some might consider early civilisation, as well as an interest in the subject of medicine, to date from around 1000 BC. However, there is evidence that well before this, the ancient Egyptians were recording details of human anatomy. There is no doubt that attempts were made to heal wounds from very early times. The practice of amputation of the nose as a punishment for sexual misdemeanours appears to date from around 3000 BC, and it has been stated that attempts were made in India to reconstruct amputated noses as early as 1500 BC. Many works on early attempts at plastic surgery mention the name of Susruta who is said to have been a Hindu surgeon born about 600 BC. Over the years I have been puzzled and then confused by varying dates, spellings and suggestions that there was no such a person but that Susruta Samhita was a compilation of works written by different authors over several centuries. Susruta (or whoever contributed to the above book) rebuilt noses with a flap of skin raised from the forehead. One thing is certain and that is the Indian surgeon was not a plastic surgeon and nor was the Italian Tagliacozzi (1530–1599), who devised a flap of arm skin to rebuild an absent nose, securing it with a complicated device. Nevertheless both names almost always appear in publications on early 'plastic surgery' as an example of early attempts at reconstructive surgery.

Between the period in which Celsus (25 BC–c.50 AD) is said to have repaired lips and ears, amongst his other interests, and the beginning of the European Renaissance (fourteenth to seventeenth century), there are few surgeons who contributed any significant advances in the field of reconstructive surgery. However, in the fifteenth century, Gustavo Branca who settled in Catania in Sicily and his son Antonio became renowned for their surgical skill. They may have been inspired by the work of Celsus and it is not known for certain how they learned nose reconstruction. Later the Vianeo family from Calabria became equally famous for their surgical work, and it is suggested that they may have been taught by the Brancas, who may have in turn inspired Tagliacozzi, the brilliant anatomist and surgeon from Bologna.

© Springer International Publishing Switzerland 2015
D. Tolhurst, *Pioneers in Plastic Surgery*, DOI 10.1007/978-3-319-19539-1_1

Perhaps the most important development in the seventeenth century was the description by William Harvey of the blood circulation and the function of the heart. But it was not until the nineteenth century that many exciting developments in the field of reconstructive surgery took place and famous names appear in our story. Amongst these are surgeons whose work has earned them a place in history and several who truly deserve the title of pioneers in plastic surgery.

Chapter 2
Nineteenth-Century Surgery

The major development during the nineteenth century was the Industrial Revolution which began in Great Britain and later spread to Europe, then Japan and America. This was a period of considerable scientific discovery and invention. Surgery was indirectly affected by two major events: Lister's introduction of antisepsis and the use of anaesthetic agents. Nitrous oxide was first used as an anaesthetic in 1844 by Wells but was replaced by Morton with the stronger agent ether in 1846. A year later, Simpson introduced chloroform which was not as popular due to the risk of cardiac complications. Surgery could now be carried out more safely, less rapidly and without causing pain to the patients. There were also valuable contributions in medicine by Pasteur, the Curies, Koch and Freud. Despite the invention of better instruments, there was however very little advance in general or plastic surgery.

There was no specialty per se of plastic surgery although Zeis had advanced the name in 1838 for the reconstructive surgery being carried out by some general surgeons. Dieffenbach was the most prolific in this field and was encouraged by Zeis to publish accounts of his work. Karl Ferdinand von Graefe, who preceded Dieffenbach at the University of Berlin, was a general surgeon and ophthalmologist but has also been described as a pioneer in plastic and reconstructive surgery. His principal contributions were in rhinoplasty, closure of cleft palates and eye surgery. He died prematurely at the age of 53 which sadly denied us further examples of his inventive mind.

Dieffenbach followed him at the Charité Hospital in Berlin, and his successor was Bernhard von Langenbeck whose chief contribution, besides his cleft palate surgery, was the introduction of resident training in general surgery. There were several other names associated with plastic surgery at this time such as Thiersch who is credited with split skin grafting and Wolfe who described the benefit of full thickness skin grafts. None of these surgeons could be described by the purist as plastic surgeons because there were no hospital appointments, societies or associations of 'plastic surgeons'. More importantly the establishment of proper training programmes as well as the foundation of scientific bodies would have to wait until the next century.

© Springer International Publishing Switzerland 2015
D. Tolhurst, *Pioneers in Plastic Surgery*, DOI 10.1007/978-3-319-19539-1_2

Chapter 3
Johann Friedrich Dieffenbach (1792–1847)

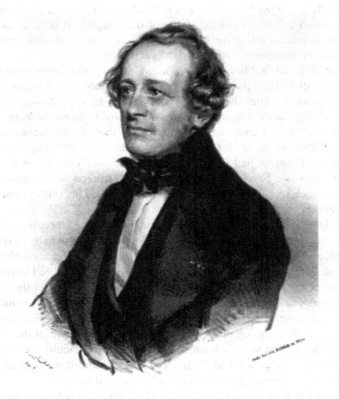

No collection of contributions to modern plastic surgery by individual surgeons would be complete without the name of Johann Dieffenbach who is considered by many to be the earliest true founder of the specialty. He was in essence a general surgeon who indeed devised and used procedures which today would fall within the ambit of plastic surgery. His publications reveal that besides plastic surgery he had

© Springer International Publishing Switzerland 2015

D. Tolhurst, *Pioneers in Plastic Surgery*, DOI 10.1007/978-3-319-19539-1_3

various other medical interests. Nevertheless, no one could hold a candle to his reconstructive contributions in the first half of the nineteenth century. However, one must not forget there were others before and after this period such as von Graefe, Langenbeck, Thiersch, Esser and Gillies who played an important role in the birth of the specialty.

Dieffenbach was born on 1 February 1892 in Konigsberg, Prussia. After the death of his father at an early age, his mother moved to her native town of Rostock where he attended school and began to briefly study theology at the University of Rostock. In 1813 he volunteered to join the army during the Napoleonic wars and was drafted as a jager (mounted hunter) until his discharge in 1815. The following year, he commenced the study of medicine in the Albertina University in Konigsberg. His participation in student political activity in Jena in 1818 as well as an unhappy love affair, despite his having attained the position of prosector, led to him leaving Konigsberg in 1920 to continue his career in Bonn. Here he worked with the surgeon and ophthalmologist Philip Franz von Walther. At this stage Dieffenbach had become interested not only in anatomy but also in surgery. It is said that he now began to demonstrate a talent for surgical techniques and made attempts to graft hairs and feathers, presumably without success.

It was now that von Walther, who introduced him to a Russian woman who was suffering from ill health, persuaded him to accompany her to Paris where he remained for 6 months. There he seized the opportunity to make the acquaintance of the celebrated Guillaume Dupuytren, Alexis de Boyer, Francois Magendie and Baron Dominique-Jean Larrey, surgeon-in-chief of the Napoleonic armies for 18 years up until Waterloo in 1815. Larrey, who was orphaned at the age of 13, was a favourite of the Emperor and distinguished himself, not only as an outstanding organiser but also as a brave man under fire as he gathered up the injured on the battlefield, so much so that the Duke of Wellington ordered his soldiers not to fire in Larrey's direction.

By 1822 Dieffenbach had returned to Germany where he became a doctor of medicine in Wurzburg. However, his peregrinations, not unusual in those days, were not at an end, and he again moved to Berlin where he married Johanna Motherby in 1824. He was appointed to the staff of the highly esteemed Charite Hospital where his reputation as a fine surgeon was enhanced by performing most of the operations for Johann Rust due to the latter's failing eyesight. In 1929 he was made chief physician to the surgical department and in 1832 became Professor Extraordinary to the University. Following the death of Karl von Graefe in 1840 at the age of 53, Dieffenbach was elected to the vacant chair at the medical faculty and became the director of the University Surgical Clinic. Von Graefe himself was a pioneer in the field of rhinoplasties, repair of the cleft palate and eyelid surgery.

It was in the latter 32 years of his life that Dieffenbach developed a strong interest in reconstructive and cosmetic surgery which were the principal subjects of his extensive contribution to the literature. Amongst other things, he wrote on blood transfusions, the relief of pain with ether, the correction of strabismus, subcutaneous tenotomies, attempts at skin grafting, wound healing and the correction of orthopaedic problems, to say nothing of the treatment of blinking and stuttering. His most impressive and memorable papers and books were those dealing with rhinoplasties and reconstructive operations throughout the body following trauma, removal of tumours and congenital deformities.

It was Eduard Zeis who introduced the term plastischen chirurgie in what can be regarded as the first real textbook of plastic surgery which was published in 1838. Zeis was inspired by the work of Dieffenbach and urged him to write the book but Dieffenbach declined. He did however write the foreword and promised to send Zeis descriptions of his new surgical work. Despite this, Zeis wrote, 'He promised so that I could include them in my book but he never got around to this, even though I made a special trip to Berlin for the purpose. And yet he kept his word for while my book was being published in Berlin he inserted whole pages containing descriptions of his most recent techniques, without showing me the manuscript beforehand'.

Zeis was born in Dresden in 1807 and was 18 years younger than Dieffenbach. He was a fine surgeon who became Professor of Surgery at Marburg before ultimately returning to Dresden where he was the chief medical officer in the new city hospital. The main interest of Zeis was collecting information on plastic surgery and its history. He rightly believed that specialisation was the key to the development and progress in the specialty.

As well as his dexterity and boldness as a surgeon, Dieffenbach had the ability to make concise and rapid decisions. He was a calm and genial person who won the affection of his students and patients alike. Strangely like von Graefe, he died whilst about to start an operation. Had he lived another 20 years, there is no doubt that he would indeed, had he followed Zeis' advice to specialise, have unquestionably deserved the title of the true founder of the specialty of plastic surgery.

In 1989 the German Society of Plastic Surgery commissioned Fritz Becker to design and produce a medal to commemorate the life and work of Dieffenbach. This has been awarded each year to surgeons worldwide who have made outstanding contributions to the specialty.

Chapter 4
Sir William Ferguson (1808–1877)

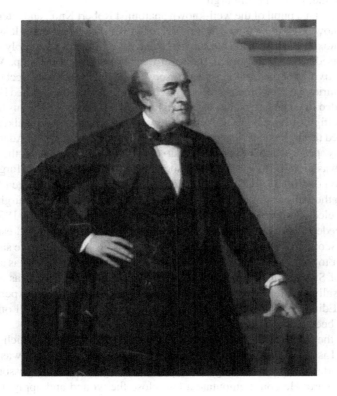

Up until the middle of the nineteenth century, general surgery consisted largely in amputations of diseased or injured limbs and lightening slash and grab raids on bladder stones. To many surgeons, these procedures, which inflicted intense pain on their patients, were abhorrent. Suddenly, in 1846, with the introduction of ether

© Springer International Publishing Switzerland 2015
D. Tolhurst, *Pioneers in Plastic Surgery*, DOI 10.1007/978-3-319-19539-1_4

anaesthesia, all this was to change and William Fergusson found himself in the happy position to benefit from the new style of surgery where pain was abolished and speed began to play a less important part in the operation. Furthermore, in place of amputations, it now became feasible to attempt surgical procedures aimed at conserving or reconstructing diseased parts, which were earlier needlessly sacrificed. It may be remembered that when Percivall Pott suffered a compound fracture of his tibia, his colleagues wished to amputate, but the timely arrival of his old teacher Edward Nourse, who thought conservative treatment feasible, saved his leg.

Fergusson coined the term 'conservative' surgery, and this aim to repair and conserve was perhaps his greatest contribution to surgery.

William Fergusson, the son of the Laird of Lochmaben, was born in Prestonpans and educated at the Lochmaben Grammar School and the High School in Edinburgh. At the age of 15, he entered a law office, but after 2 years of drudgery, he turned to the study of medicine in Edinburgh.

He was at first a pupil of the well-known anatomist Robert Knox and later consolidated his knowledge of anatomy as a prosector in Knox's department. It was to the innocent Knox that Burke had sold his first cadaver for £7, and the supply of bodies soon increased when Hare joined Burke in their notorious partnership. When the nefarious activities of these villains were discovered, Knox was the subject of embarrassing enquiries which ultimately all but cost him his life when the enraged Edinburgh rabble decided to take matters into their own hands. The mob burst into his house and burned an effigy of him, but Knox escaped by a back entrance and walked calmly, unrecognised through the thronged streets to the house of his friend Dr. Adams. Knox quite rightly protested his innocence but ever after suffered from the scandal. Fergusson was more fortunate and his association with Knox was soon forgiven.

Fergusson qualified LRCS in 1828 and, 1 year later at the tender age of 21, was admitted to the Fellowship of the Royal College of Surgeons of Edinburgh.

He was elected surgeon to the Royal Dispensary in Edinburgh in 1831 and in 1836 succeeded Liston at the Royal Infirmary where James Syme had established himself as Scotland's pre-eminent surgeon. Such was his skill that some saw in him a challenger to Syme, but 4 years later, he moved to London where he was appointed Professor of Surgery at King's College in 1840. His superlative skill as a surgeon was universally acknowledged, and the foundations for his technical expertise were laid in the Edinburgh Anatomy Department where his dissections, still on display, have never been equalled.

Prior to the first operation under ether anaesthesia in England, which was performed by Liston in December 1846, speed in the operating theatre was of paramount importance. Liston's strength and speed were legendry but Fergusson himself was no sluggard. He could amputate a leg, close the wound and apply a dressing within the space of three and a half minutes and is reputed to have once amputated at the hip-joint in 12 seconds! These heroics are now no more than history, but it must be conceded that extraordinary dexterity and an excellent knowledge of anatomy were required to reach such speed.

During operations, he expected his assistants to remain totally silent, and he never spoke, even when questions were addressed to him, until the procedure had been finished. When visitors were present, he often felt constrained to assure them that he and his assistants were on speaking terms.

Apart from his conservative approach to surgery, typified by the remark of it being 'a grand thing when by pre-science even the tip of a thumb can be saved', Fergusson also deserves mention as a pioneer in plastic surgery for the operations he performed on cleft lip and palate cases. Between 1928 and 1864, he operated on 400 cleft lips and 134 cleft palates with very few failures. What then was acclaimed as a success may nowadays be the subject of criticism, but it seems that his results were far superior to those of his contemporaries and helped to pave the way for our present techniques.

Fergusson will perhaps remain best known surgically for his maxillectomy incision and for some of the instruments, such as the lion's forceps, speculum and mouth gag, which he designed. He was an excellent carpenter and metalworker and, despite his large hands, played the violin well. He was fond of dancing Scottish reels and, like Gillies, was a keen fly fisherman. As a young man, he had married an heiress but his own labours made him a wealthy man.

In common with many great surgeons, his bedside manner left something to be desired but children seemed to adore him. He was an indifferent lecturer but wrote two surgical books: *A System of Practical Surgery* (1842) and *Progress of Anatomy and Surgery* during the twentieth century.

Honours were heaped upon him, and besides being elected to the Royal Society, he was President of the Royal College of Surgeons and President of the British Medical Association. The Prince Consort is said to have demanded of a court official: 'Supposing I had to have my leg amputated, who is the best man to do it?' 'Why Fergusson, by all means', was the reply. 'Then', said the Prince, 'he shall be my surgeon'. Fergusson was duly appointed Surgeon-in-Ordinary to Prince Albert and Surgeon-Extraordinary to Queen Victoria and was rewarded with a baronetcy in 1866.

Fergusson was tall and handsome with large dark eyes and thinning hair which gave way to baldness in later life. He had a benevolent expression and was generous and hospitable to medical students, dramatists and struggling authors, and it is perhaps to one of them that he owes this fitting epitaph: 'He had the eye of an eagle, the heart of a lion and the hand of a lady'.

Chapter 5
Twentieth-Century Surgery

The twentieth century saw the unequivocal establishment of plastic surgery as a surgical specialty, encompassing reconstructive and cosmetic operations. Societies and associations were founded, the American Society of Plastic Surgeons being the first in 1931, and then later, Vilray Blair was instrumental in the formation of the American Board of Plastic Surgery. However, close on the American's heels in 1932, the Czechoslovakian government officially recognised plastic surgery as an independent specialty which allowed Burian to employ assistants and to train them so they could be certified as specialists. Two years earlier, Charles University in Prague accepted plastic surgery as a specialty. Great Britain followed in 1946 when the first meeting of the British Association was held. Two years later, it became affiliated to the Royal College of Surgeons of England. Once proper training began, there was a rapid increase of specialists in America but a slow increase in the number of consultant plastic surgeons in Britain during the early years of the National Health Service. In the late 1960s, there were still only about 80 registered specialists, but with the increase in the population, this number has now risen to 1029.

Scientific developments, inventions, travel, communications, health and well-being have expanded far beyond those of the previous century as has plastic surgery. With the introduction of antibiotics, sophisticated local anaesthesia, the surgical microscope, computer scanning and the better understanding of diseases, all at the disposal of specialists as well as those training in the specialty, there is little wonder that there have been enormous and dramatic improvements in patient care. Two world wars produced a huge number of severe and varied injuries to stimulate the invention and skill of plastic surgeons, and many of their discoveries have formed the basis of further new ideas.

If I had to single out one field in which a really remarkable and dramatic advance was made, it would be the treatment of people who had major and often grotesque deformities of the facial skeleton. They were sometimes locked away or driven to alcoholism or drugs and often unfairly considered insane. Many were rescued from a life of misery by the work of Paul Tessier who was the undisputed founder and

© Springer International Publishing Switzerland 2015
D. Tolhurst, *Pioneers in Plastic Surgery*, DOI 10.1007/978-3-319-19539-1_5

expert of craniofacial surgery. Gillies is said to have attempted an advancement of the maxilla but found it so difficult that he gave up the idea.

I was fortunate enough to be asked to join the team when David Matthews invited Tessier to undertake the first four cases in England at the Children's Hospital at Great Ormond Street. There were so many observers in the theatre that it was necessary to relay a live video of the operation to a side room. Even then, it was not easy to understand the anatomy, and I was dispatched with a skull and some loose bones to explain exactly what was going on which seemed to be of help. Suddenly when the theatre became sparsely populated, Tessier asked where everyone had gone and on learning that I was conducting an instructive course sent for me and said: 'I didn't come here for a young man to be teaching the visitors!' Fortunately, some sort of compromise was finally reached in the coffee room.

Tessier much admired David Matthews' Bentley. At Tessier's farewell dinner, I made a short speech in which I said the team had decided to give him a Bentley, and I presented him with a splendid Matchbox model. I am glad to say we remained good friends. Later, he invited me to stay in Paris, but when I said I wanted to write about his life and career, he modestly said he didn't want anyone to do such a thing. He died in 2008 aged 90.

Besides those chosen as pioneers in the twentieth century, there have been countless other plastic surgeons who have contributed refinements and new procedures in neonatal surgery, hand surgery, congenital deformities as well as trauma and cancer cases. When my research was involved with a new idea in reconstructive work, I thought it would be the final addition to flap surgery but I was wrong of course.

Chapter 6
Robert Abbe (1851–1928)

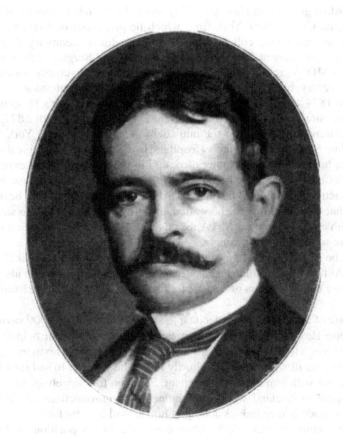

To all who practise the art and science of plastic surgery, the name of Robert Abbe will need no introduction. There are many who may have imagined, quite understandably, that Abbe was a Frenchman (a disciple perhaps of the great Victor

© Springer International Publishing Switzerland 2015

D. Tolhurst, *Pioneers in Plastic Surgery*, DOI 10.1007/978-3-319-19539-1_6

Veau) and that the family name had once been spelt with an e-acute at the end of his name. However, he was a seventh-generation American, and the e-acute had been dropped long before Robert Abbe was born in New York, the fifth of seven children.

His father was a businessman and lived in Dutch Street, New York. His mother was the daughter of William Colgate who ran a business manufacturing soap and candles also situated in Dutch Street. Later toothpaste production was added to his business, and the company was ultimately fused with Palmolive to form the famous Colgate-Palmolive Company. The family circumstances, though simple, were not altogether uncomfortable. Abbe's father was a serious and religious man who devoted much of his time and money to the sick and destitute and amongst other things founded the American Bible Union and became Governor of the New York Hospital.

Robert Abbe grew up in New York City where he attended school and later the College of the City of New York from which he graduated in 1870. For a short while, he remained on the college staff as an instructor in Geometry, English and Drawing until enrolling at the College of Physicians and Surgeons, from which he obtained his MD degree in 1874. Medical training was universally shorter in the nineteenth century, but it seemed not to the detriment of the profession.

Between 1874 and 1876, he served his internship at St. Luke's Hospital which occupied the site on the corner of 5th Avenue and 54th Street. In 1877, he was appointed Attending Surgeon to the outpatient department at New York Hospital and Attending Surgeon at St. Luke's Hospital. He next opened his surgical office on 4th Avenue, but soon after his father died, and in order to reduce his expenses, he moved his office to the family home where his sister Harriet kept house and managed his practice for him until he married. Abbe's marriage must have been a carefully calculated undertaking, for he waited until his fortieth year before stepping to the altar with a wealthy widow. Mrs Abbe possessed children from her first marriage and no more were born to the couple.

It could be said that Abbe was a true New Yorker for he lived all his life in that great city. At first after his marriage, he lived on 50th Street, where he also had his office, and for the last 8 years of his life, following his wife's death, he lived on 59th Street.

At the age of 26, Abbe wisely decided to spend some of his $1,000 savings on a trip to Europe. He had planned the venture with care and without the help of 'Europe on $5 a day (now $10 and soon perhaps $20) and hoped to spend no more than $500. His sister became ill with bronchitis shortly before he was due to sail for Liverpool and he took her with him at the last moment. So much for budgeting! Most of their time was spent in England where the kindness and introductions of Sir William McCormack made a deep impression upon him as will be seen later.

Upon his return to New York, Abbe continued in his position as Attending Surgeon at the New York Hospital until 1884 and at St. Luke's Hospital until poor health forced him to resign at the age of 73. In addition, he was Professor of Didactic

Surgery at Women's Medical College from 1878 to 1880 and lectured on surgery at the College of Physicians and Surgeons. He was Attending Surgeon at New York Babies, New York Cancer and Roosevelt Hospitals and, from 1889 until 1897, was Professor of Surgery at the New York Post-Graduate Medical College. Even at the age of 77, when he died, Abbe was still serving as Consulting Surgeon to several of his old hospitals.

From all this it may be deduced that he was a prodigious worker, and there is little wonder that his abundant publications revealed him to be possessed of an inventive streak which itself is so often the hallmark of brilliance. Nowhere is this of more value than in the field of plastic surgery, and Abbe was to turn this quality to good account in his imaginative lip switch and vaginoplasty operations.

The lip switch procedure is frequently dignified by the name of the Abbe-Estlander flap. The Finn described reconstruction of the lower lip with flaps from the upper lip as did Sabattini and Stein, but it was Abbe who, 33 years later, first used a wedge of the lower lip to correct the ugly deformity so often encountered in a repaired bilateral cleft of the upper lip. The benefits conferred by this technique are clearly visible in the drawing from Abbe's original article and the photographs of the patient on whom he first used his idea. Through this one flash of inspiration, Abbe appears to have secured for himself an immortal place in the annals of plastic surgery.

Despite the fact that McIndoe's name is sometimes coupled with the operation for an absent vagina, it was Abbe who first described the use of a split skin graft supported on a 'stuffed rubber pouch' to line a newly made vaginal cavity. An account of his first successful operation using this technique was published in 1898, the same year as his paper on the lip switch procedure appeared. Besides these two surgical discoveries, Abbe was one of the first to resect the neck of the condyle for ankylosis of the temporomandibular joint. Amongst the spectators on this occasion was Gunning, the dental surgeon who devised the oral splints which are still in use today.

Abbe was a true general surgeon with a practical interest in various reconstructive procedures. His writings and practical experience extended to abdominal and hand surgery and neurosurgery, to say nothing of the therapeutic properties of radium. It was he who brought the first radium to America in order to treat cancer and he did much to promote its use. He greatly admired the Curie's work and kept two swans, which he whimsically named Pierre and Marie, at his home in Maine. At the end of the First World War, he raised $100,000 in order to restock Madame Curie's laboratories with radium. In his 70s, Abbe suffered from aplastic anaemia, which was in all probability caused by his long exposure to radioactive elements. Earlier he had conducted experiments on himself with radium and noted reactions which varied from redness of the skin to necrosis.

Hand surgery interested him, and besides advancing a theory for the aetiology of Dupuytren's contracture, he strongly advocated fasciectomy in place of fasciotomy for this condition. The cause of cancer was also a subject upon which he exercised his mind and he indicted tobacco as a possible cause of oral cancer. Strange to say, Abbe only took up smoking at the age of 40, but perhaps this had something to do with the fact that it was also at this stage that he saddled himself with the burden of married life.

One of his notable contributions to experimental surgery was the series of operations on animals in which he successfully restored the continuity of blood vessels using glass tubing. As a further step, he divided and rejoined all the structures, except the main vessels, in the limb of a dog and was able to show that the limb survived and functioned adequately. He then postulated that it would be possible to graft back an amputated limb, but this feat was not achieved until nearly three quarters of a century later at the Massachusetts. General Hospital in Boston, during which this author was part of the anaesthetic team. Nowadays, with the help of the microscope, the replantation of digits and limbs has become commonplace.

As a teacher, he was probably at his best describing his brilliant operations in the amphitheatre where he worked, but he was an able speaker whose relaxed style also made him popular as a lecturer.

It was during his first visit to Europe that he became enchanted with the traditions of established society and, in particular, medical history and the famous contributions of great men. McCormack had shown him some of London's old institutions and took him to a memorable medical dinner at which many of the leading men in the profession were present. Later, he paid a visit to the Royal College of Physicians, where he was fascinated by a collection of instruments and other interesting objects. Amongst these was a wooden stethoscope which had belonged to Laennec, the horn of a cow which Jenner had used in his smallpox vaccination experiments and a pointer once employed by Harvey during his lectures on the circulation of the blood. Later, as a result of this experience, he set out to acquire some interesting belongings of Lord Lister, Jenner, Pasteur and Curie which were ultimately housed in the cabinet of the College of Physicians in Philadelphia where he founded the Custodianship of Rush. History had cast its spell upon him, and he later observed 'There are some names in our profession... whose very spirit evokes a thrill when we come into actual touch with their belongings...'.

As well as medical history, the Red Paint Indians of the Cadillac Mountains fascinated him, and it was on frequent trips to Maine where he had a house at Brook End that he studied these members of the Appalachian Tribe. He also assembled stone-age relics which were discovered on Mount Desert in Maine and founded a museum, which bears his name, in Lafayette National Park to house them.

His more mundane hobbies included cycling, billiards, chess and baseball. Painting, photography and model making also occupied his leisure hours. He frequently made use of plaster of Paris in his work to demonstrate deformities. In fact, one can see models of hands made by Abbe illustrating a lobster claw deformity and Dupuytren's contracture, in a photograph taken by him of the painter J.W. Alexander. Alexander was a close friend who had painted a portrait of Abbe's sister Helen, and it was through this friendship that Abbe developed his interest in painting. His watercolour portraits and pictures of his garden, showing the flowers which he loved, are by no means inconsiderable works of art. Abbe was one of the early proponents of the use of photography for medical documentation, and he was an eager experimenter with colour and flash photography.

It was in later life that Abbe became aware of an increasing tightness of his hat, the classic warning sign of Paget's disease, and his fears were confirmed by an X-ray examination made in London. However, his spirit was not daunted, and even when overtaken by aplastic anaemia, he remained the same friendly, charming figure which had endeared him to so many throughout his long and busy life.

Chapter 7
Jacques Joseph (1865–1934)

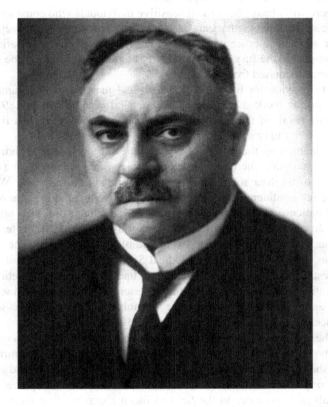

Jacob Levin Joseph was born in Konigsberg, Prussia, on 6 September 1865, but the city's name is now no more than a spectre, which rises from the mists of history, for it was renamed Kaliningrad in 1945, when it was ceded to the Soviet Union. Joseph was the youngest of three children, and his father, Israel Joseph, was a Rabbi who naturally brought his offspring up according to the Jewish faith.

© Springer International Publishing Switzerland 2015
D. Tolhurst, *Pioneers in Plastic Surgery*, DOI 10.1007/978-3-319-19539-1_7

At the age of 14, young Jacques Joseph, as he later preferred to be known, was sent to the Sophien Gymnasium in Berlin to further his education. After his schooling had been completed, he embarked on the study of medicine at the Friedrich Wilhelm University in Berlin, from which he received a certificate in 1890. This was not a formal M.D. degree, but according to his widow, his M.D. was granted by the University of Leipzig. Unfortunately, it has never been possible to resolve the question of the origin of his degree, since part of the archives at Leipzig were destroyed during the Second World War.

For a short while, following graduation, Joseph worked with Neumann at the Children's Clinic in Berlin, before setting up in private practice in 1891. One year later, he became an assistant to Professor Julius Wolff at the University Orthopaedic Clinic in Berlin. In 1896, to the surprise, nay, horror, of the hospital dignitaries, word reached them that Joseph had apparently taken leave of his senses and operated upon a small boy to correct his protruding ears!

In life, there will always be some insensitive individuals who consider the common facial features, such as 'bat ears', to be of no significance, but Joseph and his little patient were of another persuasion. Despite a scientific publication on his method of otoplasty, the fury of the university committee was not to be assuaged, and Joseph was dismissed from his post.

In order to provide for his family (Joseph had married in 1893 and had one daughter Bella), he worked for 2 years as a general practitioner. In 1898, his life changed as the result of the visit of a young man who asked Joseph if he could reduce his large and ugly nose!

Far from daunted by the ruins of his academic career, Joseph withdrew to the serenity of the morgue, where he worked out a plan of campaign upon a cadaver's nose, ignorant of the four stage nasal correction already published by Weir. Eight days later, he felt confident enough to put his operative technique to the test on the hawk-nosed patient, who not only survived the experiment but also appeared as delighted as Joseph with the result. Joseph was moved to publish this technique in the same year, and so the foundations were laid of his future fame. The successful operation was reported to the Berlin Medical Society in May 1898, and from then on, his interests began to centre more and more upon corrective 'cosmetic' surgery. It was not until 1904 that he reported his experience with intranasal incisions for rhinoplasty, and 1 year later, he was able to publish an account of his technique, which had been used with success on more than 100 patients.

By now, he had achieved an international reputation upon which he continued to build until the outbreak of the First World War. The flood of facial injuries consequent upon the vicious trench warfare soon began to occupy him, and in 1916, a special unit for plastic surgery at the Charite Hospital in Berlin was placed under his care. His skill and ingenuity in the field of facial reconstruction were ultimately rewarded in 1919 with the title of professor. Joseph continued at the Charite until 1921 when he resigned and devoted himself entirely to private practice.

There was intense rivalry in the field of private practice in Berlin at this time, but despite the fact that many surgeons thought nasal surgery was simple, Joseph rose above his colleagues and in the early 1920s was predominant in his specialty. Professor Axhausen, who had watched him operate, agreed that the surgical technique was not difficult but, nevertheless, it took Joseph to get a really good result.

Strangely enough, there were three Professor Josephs all working in Berlin at the same time, and the public is supposed to have distinguished between the three by applying the first letter of each one's specialty to the individual name. Thus, the gastroenterologist (Magenkrankheiten) became Moseph; the dermatologist (Hautkrankheiten), Hoseph; and the nasal expert, Noseph!

The vagaries of the public, however, were equalled if not excelled by Joseph himself. For some years, he refused to use rubber gloves whilst operating and instead wore rubber fingerstalls on his thumb, index and middle fingers, as he considered touch to be of paramount importance. He did not favour cap nor mask, and it was as though he believed his thick moustache and the observation of silence in the theatre to be adequate for the prevention of infection. Nearly 80 years after his death, a careful study has revealed him to be correct in his assumption.

His taciturnity did not endear him to those attending his so-called courses on nasal surgery, for which privilege the participants were obliged to part with a considerable sum of money. Safian has given a nice account of the situation: 'The 10 day course consisted merely of permission to observe his operations. He made no comments and did not describe the various steps of his rhinoplastic technique'. It was only later that he was persuaded by Safian, himself, later to achieve world renown in the same field of surgery to improve the 'course' by including a combined anatomical and surgical programme on the cadaver.

Outside the operating room, Joseph could also assume the mantle of arrogance. Esser found this disagreeable, and when asked by Safian if he spoke English, Joseph replied (in German): 'It is beneath my dignity'. On the whole, however, he was kind and polite to his patients but correct, though strict, with his staff. For a while, Aufricht and Coelst worked with him as assistants, and he regularly attracted visitors throughout Germany and abroad.

As a surgeon, Joseph appeared to operate with ease despite the careful planning and measurements, which preceded his operations. The importance of handling the tissues with delicacy was something not lost on Joseph, who referred to this as 'biologic sense'. At the same time, his meticulous preparations and familiar routine eliminated all but the necessary operative steps, many of which he accompanied by the utterance of the word 'so'. He did not confine himself to nasal surgery, and besides his work on war victims, he performed facelifts, ear corrections, breast reduction and chin augmentations. For the latter and also for building up the nasal skeleton, he was in the habit of using carved ivory, which he obtained from a piano factory. The source of his supply, he refused to reveal to Safian, because he said 'You Americans buy up everything with your dollars and make things expensive for us'. Whether or not Joseph's economic theories were sound or merely anachronistic is open to debate, but it must be admitted that such remarks of late have been heard to come from the lips of supposed experts in the field of economics.

To those who criticised him as a 'cosmetic surgeon', one can answer that his main aim was to make his patients inconspicuous and in this, he usually succeeded, as his results were often described as natural looking.

Most well-known surgeons have designed instruments, and Joseph had a special one for nearly every step in his rhinoplasties, many of which are still popular throughout the world. Nowadays, the description of his first rhinoplasty seems crude, but later Joseph changed his technique, which closely resembles that practised by many modern surgeons.

Writing was an aspect of his work which Joseph did not neglect, and he left behind many papers, mostly on nasal surgery and an excellent book *Nasenplastik und sonstige Gesichtsplastik*. He was fond of coining new words from Greek or Latin, but few, if any, have survived him.

Nowadays, as a rule, it is frowned upon to rush into print on the strength of one successful case, but this is exactly what Joseph did following his first ear and nose corrections. Even so, he was to be disappointed if he thought that the account of his maiden rhinoplasty was the first of its kind, for Weir in America could rightly claim priority by a few months. But, undaunted, Joseph dissected Weir's operation, step by step, and concluded that the only similarities between the two were a reduction in the size of the noses and the desire of both surgeons to improve the psychological state of their patients.

As Aufricht has observed, 'Priority was and apparently always will be an important ambition of surgeons'. Joseph's technique was undoubtedly original in that in one operation, he achieved what Weir accomplished in four. Important though this may have been to Joseph himself, what matters now is that the man's genius has been recognised by those following him, and Aufricht's epithet of 'the world's unchallenged father of modern rhinoplastic surgery' is well deserved.

If often he was uncivil during his working hours, his friends and family saw him in a different light. His warmth and humour made him popular, especially amongst women in society, but his wife commanded his true affection. For many years, she assisted him in his practice, and her delicate features and striking profile were an inspiration to Joseph as he records in his book on rhinoplasty.

Having recovered from the financial losses, which many incurred during the Great War, Joseph began construction of a palatial villa (complete with lift) in 1924. He is said to have implanted a bottle containing the following verse in the concrete foundations during the construction:

Und deckt mich einst der grune Rasen,
so wisest, dies war gebaut von Nasen.

And one day as I'm covered with the green lawn
Know that his house was built from noses

His holidays were often spent at Karlsbad in Czechoslovakia, where he went to relax and take the waters as did many of the well-to-do in an attempt to 'cleanse their bodies' and throw off their ailments. Joseph loved fine food, and it is no wonder that his large and imposing figure ran to fat for his only hobbies seemed to have been the collecting of paintings, woodcuts and ivory figures! In his youth, he had been a competent artist and flirted briefly with sculpturing.

In later years, during the rise of the Nazi party, Joseph's reputation protected him against persecution, but one of his secretaries, Fraulein Wittig, began to blackmail him. She took down his conversations and reported them to party officials so that Joseph was finally arrested and interrogated but happily released.

One winter's morning in 1934, he was struck down by a heart attack in the hall of his house, where he died immediately. His daughter and son-in-law fled to Nice in 1934, and 4 years later, his wife joined them there. In 1941, she made her way via Spain, Portugal and Cuba to America, where for many years she lived in San Francisco.

Chapter 8
Otto Lanz (1865–1935)

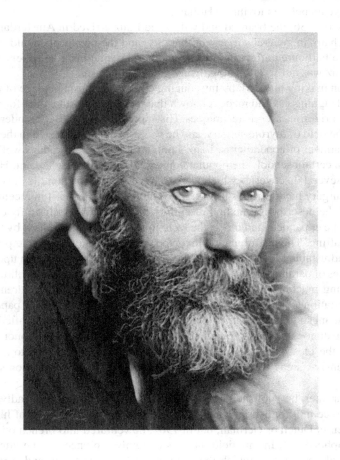

D. Tolhurst, *Pioneers in Plastic Surgery*, DOI 10.1007/978-3-319-19539-1_8

Until the outbreak of the Second World War, there was a very considerable German influence on the development of medicine in Holland. This was particularly evident in the field of surgery where in Utrecht, for example, the Chair of Surgery was successively occupied by three of Billroth's pupils from Vienna. The first of these incumbents was Salzer (1890–1893); the second, Freiherr Von Einelsbert (1893–1896); and the third, Narath (1896–1906). During these times, the average Dutch medical students' bookshelves would have been largely filled with German textbooks.

The appointment of Otto Lanz to the Chair of Surgery in Amsterdam in 1902 was no exception to this trend for his education had been decidedly Germanic. Lanz was born in Steffisburg in Switzerland in 1865 and later studied at the Universities of Geneva, Bern, Basle and Leipzig. He completed his surgical training under the renowned Theodor Kocher (1841–1917) in Bern, and it was in this city that he practised for 8 years before moving to Holland.

At the age of 36, the bearded and wild-eyed Lanz arrived in Amsterdam. There were two chairs in general surgery in that city, and the occupants could hardly be said to have harboured affection for one another. Despite his good scientific background, Lanz was not welcomed with any great enthusiasm.

He began making his mark by introducing ether anaesthesia in place of the more unreliable laughing gas and made it known that there was no substitute for anything but the most rigorous aseptic techniques. His apprenticeship in Bern rendered him a master in the field of thyroid surgery, and he was especially interested in the prostate and the treatment of appendicitis. Lanz's point, though not nowadays well known, was once in certain schools the popular equivalent of McBurney's point. His publications of several discoveries which were to have an influence on the development of plastic surgery have perhaps been somewhat neglected, at least in recent times.

In 1907, he described a method of cutting holes in a Thiersch graft so that the graft could be expanded, and this is the technique which we now know by the name of mesh grafting. The instrument he invented consisted of a sort of stamp in which was fixed adjustable knives, and when the apparatus was pressed down upon a skin graft, a series of parallel cuts were made. He named the device a Hautschlittsapparat, a skin-slitting machine. Lanz came upon the idea when he saw children at play, making imitation concertinas by snipping parallel slits in strips of paper. Lanz intended the mesh to be used in two pieces – one for the area being grafted and the other for the donor site. It was principally to hasten the healing of the donor area that he devised the idea, but he pointed out that the mesh could be used to advantage where extensive areas were to be grafted or if the amount of donor skin was limited.

One year later, he published a German version of the article but, sadly, did not see fit to grace the English language with a paper on his idea. Most of his papers were written in Dutch or German, but in 1902, he ventured into French on the subject of lymphoedema. In this field, he was certainly a pioneer for he attempted a physiological operation in which the deep fascia was fenestrated and strips of the fascia threaded into the bone marrow cavity. He published several other articles in Dutch and wrote extensively on free skin grafting.

Upon the outbreak of the First World War in 1914, Holland, as did Switzerland, declared itself neutral. As a Swiss citizen, domiciled in Holland, it was thus natural that he should offer his services to the German wounded, on purely humanitarian grounds. Quite a number of Dutch did the same, amongst whom were Esser (1877–1946) who had originally studied in Brunn (now Brno) and Henri Rath, who had worked in Paris with Tuffier.

Lanz became consultant surgeon to the field hospital in Trier, and he described his wartime experiences in the Dutch Medical Journal in 1915. Later, in 1931, he acted as V.M.E. Winters' promoter for his thesis on 'War and Surgery'.

Lanz, who, it will be remembered, was a fierce proponent of scrupulous asepsis, realised the dangers of the indifferent dressing techniques which were in operation on the battlefields at the beginning of the 1914–1918 War. His first-hand experience as head of the Dutch Red Cross ambulance service confirmed his anxiety, and he drew attention to the inadequate number of medical orderlies and the poor early treatment of wounds which in turn had an important influence on the long-term prognosis of the wounded. Most of the wounded he observed soon became seriously infected, and he attributed this in some degree to the bad hygiene in the trenches.

He had the idea of fitting out a special automobile in which laparotomies could be undertaken. In fact, these were variations on the 'ambulance volantes' introduced by Larrey, Napoleon's military surgeon. As the war became bogged down, these 'automobile chirurgicales' were slowly adopted, and the good results proved their need and value. Thus, stepwise, the horse-drawn vehicles of Larrey led via the laparotomy ambulances of Lanz to today's helicopter service, all of which coupled the advantages of rapid transport with early treatment. Thanks to the efficient evacuation of the severely wounded, great strides were made in the field of plastic surgery. But for this, the victims of many reparable jaw and skin defects would have perished.

Otto Lanz was an enthusiastic art collector and listed many artists amongst his acquaintances. The Swiss painter, Ferdinand Hodler, persuaded him to don the uniform of a lancer in which he painted Lanz holding a halberd. Many generations of medical students will have felt the stern gaze of Lanz upon them during their surgical lectures in the old Binnengasthuis in Amsterdam, and not a few of them, including this author, will have been ignorant of the fact that the bearded face peering out at them from Jan Toorop's portrait is that of Otto.

Holland's most famous writer, Simon Vestdijk, unmistakably portrays him as Lenz, a professor of surgery who speaks bad Dutch, liberally sprinkled with Germanisms. In Vestdijk's book *The Last Chance*, Anton Wachter is really the author himself who is subjected to a gruelling examination by the forbidding Lenz. As already mentioned, there were two chairs of surgery in Amsterdam, and so long as the students were examined by the professor with whom they had spent their surgical assistantship, all went well. Woe betide the unfortunate student who by misadventure fell into the hands of the opposition, as it were. In the book, Anton Wachter is directed to the wrong professor but is happily rescued from his ordeal in the nick of time by a secretary.

Lanz considered teaching as an important part of his duties, and he never missed his lectures which were extremely well attended. Besides their scientific content, his lectures were sprinkled with amusing and philosophical remarks as well as observations on subjects of topical interest.

His parries and the thrusts of his colleagues in the literature in the same concise and philosophical fashion and his writings in the Dutch Medical Journal are still a pleasure to read.

All Lanz's students were treated correctly but at the same time were subjected to the strictest of discipline, for which most were later grateful. Alas! How things have changed. Despite his forbidding sternness, he had a soft heart for his patients and was a dedicated lover of the arts. These conflicting facets of character served to enhance his personality and never came between him and his work.

Chapter 9
Erich Lexer (1867–1937)

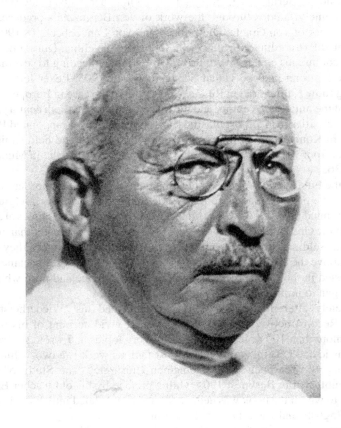

© Springer International Publishing Switzerland 2015
D. Tolhurst, *Pioneers in Plastic Surgery*, DOI 10.1007/978-3-319-19539-1_9

Lexer was born in Freiburg, Germany, on 22 May 1867, the son of a Professor of German Languages. By the age of nine, he was already showing talent for art and started a course in modelling, sculpturing and painting with a professional sculptor.

Painting and drawing of plaster figures and muscle men converted him to anatomy, and it was but a short step further to the study of medicine. During his medical studies, he was much impressed by a hand operation which was being performed by Herman Maas, the successor to Ernst von Bergmann in Wurzberg, and from this moment, Lexer decided to become a surgeon.

Lexer wrote his thesis in 1890 in Wurzberg and became an instructor in anatomy in 1891–1892 in Merkel's anatomical institute in Gottingen. In 1892, he moved to Berlin as a surgical resident in the surgical clinic of Ernst von Bergmann, who was a very good teacher and a successful surgeon, researcher and writer. This second surgical clinic of Berlin (II. Chirurgischen Klinink der Universitat Berlin) had become extremely famous through the work of von Bergmann's predecessors, as well as the work of von Graefe, Diefferbach and von Langenbeck. In 1902, Lexer was appointed Extraordinary Professor in Surgery at the clinic. During this period, there were continuous clinches with Prof. von Bergmann leading to several clashes between both strong and individual personalities. In 1905, Lexer left Berlin for Konigsberg (now Kaliningrad in Russia). As was often the case in Europe during the latter part of the nineteenth century and the first part of the twentieth century, Lexer's peripatetic activities read almost like those of a nomad. He was appointed Professor of Surgery in Konigsberg (Kaliningrad) from 1905 to 1910 and held similar positions in Jena from 1911 to 1916, in Freiburg from 1919 to 1928 and in Munich from 1928 to 1936.

During the First World War, Lexer held the rank of Admiral in the German Navy. At this time, he organised a centre for Plastic Surgery in Flanders (Belgium), and later he continued his work on the victims of trench warfare in the clinics at Jena and Freiburg. In the Great War, the carnage and misery were much greater than may now be imagined. Soldiers suffered the most appalling facial wounds when they exposed their head above the trenches to the enemy fire. Like Gillies, Lexer became particularly interested in the reconstructive surgery of the jaw, face and nose which, little by little, began to improve the lot of these wretched cases.

Immediately after the war, in 1918, he published his 'Wiederherstellungschirurgie' (Reconstructive Surgery) which gives a vivid account of his work. He published more than 100 articles on plastic surgery topics and wrote several books on both plastic and general surgery. His most famous work is a two-volume handbook of surgery 'Lehrbuch der Allgemeinen Chirurgie' (The Study of General Surgery), published in Berlin in 1904, with a preface by his old teacher Ernst von Bergmann, to whom the book was dedicated. It was translated into many languages, including English, and went through 20 editions.

Lexer was a large man of great physical strength who abhorred weakness of any sort. His favourite sports were rowing and early morning horse rides. He loved sunbathing and his closely shaved head was always well tanned! He was a typical Bavarian with a passion for driving fast and expensive motorcars, and he had a weakness for Mercedes-Benz models. His Maybach 12 would, nowadays, be worth a fortune! He even conducted examinations whilst polishing his beloved cars. On special occasions, he was fond of wearing the Bavarian national dress, the 'Lederhose', which includes a pair of leather shorts complete with supporting shoulder straps. Amongst his less rumbustious hobbies, painting and sculpturing still played an important part in his leisure hours.

National and international contacts with renowned colleagues were legion. His discussions with the gentle, philosophic August Bier became legendary in Germany, but Lexer, always an extrovert, was apt to lose control of himself and become too heated. As a result, they avoided one another for a long period in their private lives.

Another of Lexer's renowned antagonists was the Frenchman Victor Veau, who was a recognised authority in the field of cleft lip and palate surgery. According to Lexer, Veau's method worked only for Frenchmen, since they speak with the mouth, but not for the Germans who have a more guttural speech from the throat. Lexer expended much time and space on roundly condemning Veau's method. In return, Veau sent him an autographed copy of his 'Division Palatine' and invited Lexer to see the operations for himself in the Paris clinic where he worked. Lexer's refusal was short and sharp: 'I shall not cross the Rhine'. However, when Veau extended a personal invitation to Mrs. Lexer and their two daughters to enjoy the delights of Paris, Lexer swallowed his words and decided to accompany the ladies!

In 1932, the Lexers arrived in France and were cordially received. Despite the obvious language barrier, Lexer himself enjoyed his stay and even operated with Veau. The following year when Veau returned the visit, he even found Lexer using his technique which he had once so fiercely condemned. Lexer travelled widely and, besides several visits to Spain, was a guest of Stewart Halsted in America. As a lecturer, he was much in demand, and his interest ranged over many subjects, but plastic surgery was his special hobby. He spoke regularly on the treatment of burns, free transplantation, arthroplasty and mammoplasty. His lectures were clear and scientific and accompanied by profuse and skilfully executed drawings on the blackboard. When he operated, Lexer's elegant style resembled the beautiful movements of a sculptor. Great though he was, there were flaws in his character, and his authoritative manner at times degenerated to painful bluntness or extraordinary rudeness. Yet he could demonstrate seductive charm, and underneath it, there seemed to beat a warm heart.

In 1937, his robust health and vitality began to wane. He went to Berlin for a medical check-up which was performed by von Bergmann's son, but this revealed no serious problem. After returning to his hotel, he telephoned his wife to tell her the good news, but he collapsed in the telephone booth and died instantly of a myocardial infarction on 4 December 1937.

During his life, through his many books, articles, lectures and training of young surgeons, Lexer was really the driving force behind the development of modern German plastic surgery.

Chapter 10
Hippolyte Morestin (1869–1919)

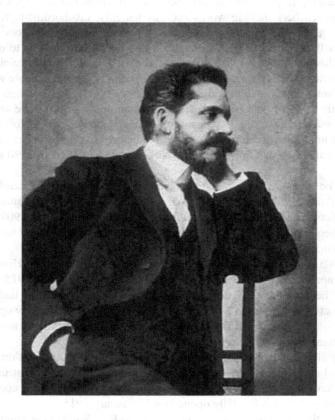

Hippolyte Morestin was born on 1 September 1869 in the town of Basse-Pointe on the small island of Martinique which lies north of St. Lucia and Barbados in the Eastern Caribbean. It was here on the 8 May 1902 at 8 o'clock in the morning that the Mount Pelee volcano, which had lain dormant for some years, erupted. Ten days

© Springer International Publishing Switzerland 2015

D. Tolhurst, *Pioneers in Plastic Surgery*, DOI 10.1007/978-3-319-19539-1_10

before the eruption, many inhabitants had left the city due to some rumblings and clouds of smoke emitted from the volcano. Within 1 min following the eruption, the neighbouring city of Saint Pierre was completely engulfed in a cloud of ash, steam and dust which reached a temperature of 1075° centigrade. All but two of the remaining 30,000 inhabitants were killed, and their buildings and belongings totally destroyed. Amongst the victims of the disaster was a well-to-do and highly respected surgeon, Dr. Charles Amédée Morestin, along with 21 of his relatives. Fortunately, one of his sons Hippolyte Morestin and his brother Amédée had both been sent to France to study. Their father had also studied and worked in France where he was a prosector of anatomy and an ancient intern in Besancon. In addition, he presented his doctoral thesis to the Faculty of Medicine of Paris in 1862.

The circumstances surrounding Hippolyte's departure were not altogether pleasant for he had been expelled from the Seminary College of Saint Pierre owing to his very poor academic performance and extremely difficult personality. Comments made by his teachers include words such as naughty, insubordinate, rebellious, quarrelsome and lazy, scarcely those one would associate with someone destined for such a brilliant career. His father had then dispatched him to Paris to undertake more disciplined schooling. Once this was completed, he apparently celebrated by promptly burning all his papers despite having obtained his baccalaureate with ease.

His first intention was to become a naval officer, and despite a longing for his distant family and early island life beside the ocean, his poor physique and fragile personality made a seafaring career impossible, and he decided to follow in the footsteps of his father and brother to study medicine. He passed his examinations without difficulty and was appointed intern of Hospitals of Paris in 1890 at the age of 21.

In 1904, he became a Surgery Associate and, in 1905, an honorary member of the Society of Anatomy. There followed many communications to the anatomy and surgery societies, and he was elected to full membership on 22 May 1907. He also became a member of the Societies of Dermatology and Syphiligraphy to which he contributed many reviews in Paris and elsewhere in France.

From 1905, he was very busy as a surgeon in the Saint Antoine Hospital, the Hospital Tenon from 1911 and finally the Hospital Saint Louis from 1915 where he became the head of the ENT department. Now at the age of 36, he had become highly respected and began to attract universal interest. He had already operated at the International Congress of Surgery in New York in 1914 and from now on was visited by many foreign colleagues who had come to Paris.

Not long after the outbreak of the First World War in 1914, he was drafted into the army and appointed to the Val de Grace Hospital where he was entrusted with the care of severe facial injuries. There he organised the centre for reconstructive facial surgery which was formally opened on 15 January 1915.

It is interesting to note that at the outbreak of the First World War, many inhabitants who felt proud to fight for their 'motherland' of France volunteered for the army and were sent to the front. The fighting on the European continent lays some 7,000 km away, and little did those who were sent there know what awaited them! Of the 8,788 inhabitants who served on the front, 1,876 lost their lives. As the war developed, the flow of injured French soldiers steadily increased, and by August 1919, Morestin was responsible for no less than 480 beds! By 1916, the numbers were too great for the Val de Grace, and Morestin was appointed chief surgeon to the face and jaw unit at the Hospital Rothschild. Unfortunately, he was not in favour of the wide use of prostheses employed by the dentists as he preferred reconstructive surgery for facial defects, refusing to accept dentists as equals. He called them mechanics who were only to be at his beck and call as he needed. When Morestin decided to leave the hospital, despite the intervention of the American ambassador, no successor could be found, and the unit was closed.

In June 1915, Gillies, who was then an ENT surgeon in London, went on leave to Paris where he visited Morestin who he heard was performing amazing operations to reconstruct the face and jaws of patients following cancer and war injuries. Morestin received him courteously and allowed him to watch the removal of an extensive cancerous growth on the face with a deftness and skill that held him spellbound, especially when Morestin then proceeded to close the resultant defect with a large flap of skin from the neck. Gillies is reputed to have said 'I fell in love with the work on the spot'. Later he wrote that 'this was the work I wanted to do', and so was born the founder of modern British plastic surgery.

Much has been written of Morestin's fierce and fractious personality and his strange moods. Some have described him as dark and reclusive, but there is little doubt that the loss of his family in the terrible volcanic disaster must have had some effect upon him. Perhaps the fact that he was a Creole may have also played a part. An example of his unpredictable behaviour is the occasion of Gillies' second visit to him at the Val de Grace Hospital. He was refused entry to Morestin's operating theatre, and when Gillies produced his official French permit, Morestin shrugged his shoulders, turned away and disappeared behind closed doors.

It is strange that no one has pointed out that the brief acquaintance of these two men was however responsible for a remarkable change in both the recognition of their names and fame and the development of the specialty of plastic surgery. Nearly every biographical publication about Gillies mentions his visit to Morestin whose name has become famous as a result. Very little had ever been published about Morestin's life and contributions to surgery until papers by Lalardrie (1972) and Blair (1982) attracted attention. Now his name ranks highly amongst the pioneers. After Gillies' visit to Morestin, he decided to give up ENT surgery in favour of plastic surgery in which his name has become a byword in this subject, to say nothing of his influence on many of the principles of plastic surgery.

Those who watched him operating were all impressed with his knowledge of anatomy and the speed and accuracy of Morestin's dissections, especially in the neck. Prior to his work with the war injuries, it is evident that he was a tireless worker, and it seems he had no other interests in life beyond his career. He was principally an ENT surgeon, much occupied with radical surgery for cancer of the face, tongue, jaw and pharyngeal area which led to his expertise in neck dissections.

Morestin was also busy with surgery beyond the head and neck, in which he advocated the importance of good aesthetic results, especially in the breast. He undertook various cosmetic operations such as the correction of prominent ears, breast reductions and face lifts. Besides the various skin flaps, which he preferred to skin grafts if possible, he was the first or one of the earliest advocates of cartilage grafts. Amongst the eminent patients who sought his opinion during his visit to New York was Sarah Bernhardt who had broken her right knee when she leaped from the parapet in the closing stages of Tosca. The wound never healed properly and her leg was finally amputated above the knee. Morestin also had the dubious distinction of being consulted by Al Capone at this time.

In all, during his relatively short working life, he published the astonishing number of 634 papers and various communications in French. As a result, it seems as if scarcely any of his writing was read in the English-speaking countries, and this is the main reason why his work was not well known until the First World War. Many English and American surgeons were present in France, but within a year of the end of the war, Morestin was dead. Moreover, according to Lalardrie, Morestin wrote too many papers and not enough books.

There is universal agreement that Morestin was a skilful and very experienced surgeon. In addition, he was also an extremely knowledgeable anatomist, and this enabled him to perform his dissections with confidence and speed. He had long, slender fingers, but it is not the shape of one's fingers but the way in which they are used that makes for skilful surgery. McIndoe's fingers were likened to sausages but he was a very deft craftsman! Duhamel who worked with Morestin described the 'extreme elegance of his surgery' which however could suddenly become wild and ferocious.

He was of average height, slim and frail and walked with a slow and slight stoop. Photographs of him reveal his dark, short cropped hair, a pointed goatee beard and full moustache as well as dark and piercing eyes. Mention has been made of his sensitive and labile character. Although described as kind and big hearted, he found it difficult to accept contradiction and criticism. Early on he probably suffered from tuberculosis, and his tireless devotion to work no doubt undermined his frail health still further. He died aged 49 of a pulmonary complication during the Spanish flu epidemic in 1919. One of the main streets in Basse-Pointe, his birth place, is named after him. The nurses who worked with him spoke with admiration of his skill as well as his sacrificial devotion to patients. Both nurses and patients attended his funeral and followed him on foot to his final resting place in Paris. There can be little better than this as an epitaph.

We know nothing of this lonely man's private life in Paris, where he lived, who if any were his friends and whether he eschewed the delights of the opera, theatre, restaurants and the company of women in the great and exciting city. It seems that work and little else interested him. He has been variously described as an anatomist, general surgeon, ENT surgeon and then latterly a maxillofacial surgeon but, most of all, a true plastic surgeon.

Chapter 11
Vilray P. Blair (1811–1955)

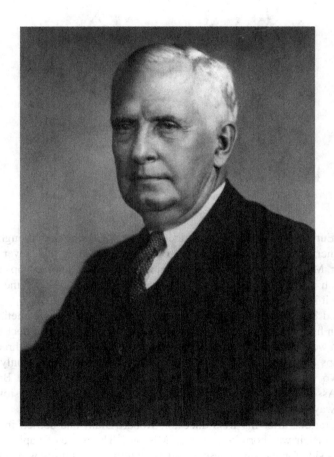

© Springer International Publishing Switzerland 2015
D. Tolhurst, *Pioneers in Plastic Surgery*, DOI 10.1007/978-3-319-19539-1_11

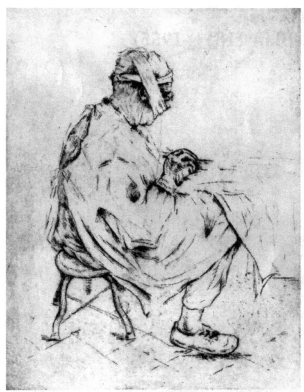

A Note on a surgeon   Gertrude Hance

When two European plastic surgery residents were asked who they thought was the greatest American plastic surgeon, they confessed that they had never heard of Vilray Blair. Mention of the Blair knife soon rectified this temporary lapse of memory, but such a story emphasises how our working span and any fame that may accompany it is so short-lived.

Blair died 8 years after retiring from active practice and was something of an exception in his field, for he spent 54 years of his life working as a doctor, the last 30 of which were devoted almost exclusively to plastic surgery. These three decades were perhaps the most formative in modern plastic surgery for not only did they embrace two world wars but they also saw the establishment of the British and American Associations of Plastic Surgery several years after Czechoslovakia had shown the way in this field.

Six generations after his Irish ancestor, Robert Blair, had settled in America, Vilray Papin Blair was born in St. Louis, Missouri. The name of Papin came from his mother's side for she was a descendant of an immigrant family which had come to New Orleans from France. Blair's maternal grandfather, Dr. Timothy Papin, was a distinguished gynaecologist who had studied in Paris and on one occasion acted as interpreter for Sir James Simpson when he introduced chloroform anaesthesia to the continent.

At the time of Blair's childhood, the population of America was less than 65 million and he wrote that his school was largely surrounded by open countryside. He and his chums rode to school on horseback and often went hunting on their way home. He grew up in St. Louis, beside the muddy Mississippi, and obtained his B.A. at Christian Brothers College. In 1890, he embarked on the study of medicine at St. Louis Medical College where he claimed Gray's Anatomy was the only textbook he possessed.

After 1 year at medical school, he went out west to erect telephone wires in the Colorado Rockies and, upon his return to St. Louis, toyed with the idea of studying electrical engineering in place of medicine, but his father persuaded him to finish his degree which he did in 1893. It can be seen that medical schooling could be completed with dispatch in those days. A period of 2-year internship at the Mullanphy Hospital in St. Louis was then succeeded by a post as instructor in practical anatomy at Washington University also in St. Louis.

For the next 18 years, Blair taught anatomy and surgery at Washington University where he introduced the use of modelling clay for the study of anatomy, which in 1906 led to the publication of his first book *A Textbook for the Modelling of Human Bones in Clay*. This thorough grounding and interest in anatomy undoubtedly contributed to his surgical skill, as well as his inventive reconstructive finesse. It will perhaps be remembered that many fine surgeons during the nineteenth century devoted some hours each day to dissecting the cadaver; Sir Astley Cooper, for example, rose at six each morning and dissected till eight when he ate a simple breakfast and then proceeded to the hospital. He even had a dissecting room built in his summer home, for to him, a day without dissecting was anathema. Blair's interest in anatomy, however, was less passionate.

In his 20s, Blair's heart was not altogether devoted to the practice or at least the conventional practice of medicine. From 1894 he spent about 5 years associated in practice with Dr. Tupper, at the end of which he gave up his association and decided to go to sea. Now he 'found out that life was really worth living'. Many will subscribe to the sentiments of Dr. Johnson who considered a ship in most respects to be far less agreeable than that of a prison. However, Blair was only enticed back home by the entreaties of his family.

It was after recuperating in Italy from an illness that he served on various tramps in the Mediterranean and later travelled to Scotland where he entered the Edinburgh Medical School. The Boer War was in progress, and Blair decided to apply for a post as surgeon on a British ship but was turned down as he had none of his diplomas with him. Out of money, he pawned his watch chain, a family heirloom, and then took a job as surgeon on a ship sailing to Para near the mouth of the Amazon. The accounts of his adventures as ship's surgeon on the South America run, to say nothing of a trip to the coast of West Africa, the 'white man's graveyard' and a stint as troop-ship surgeon during the Ashanti War, read, as Webster observed, like a tale from Joseph Conrad. Beriberi, smallpox, yellow fever and malaria took the place of today's seasickness and sunburn on tropical cruises.

Upon his return to St. Louis at the age of 30, just after the turn of the century, Blair wanted to go into business with his father who again persuaded him to return to medicine. At 36, he married Kathryn Johnson, whose private income kept the growing family's body and soul together, as he was not yet making enough to support his wife and children.

Matters took a turn for the better when he was offered a partnership by Bartlett, and besides appointments to the visiting staff at St. Luke's and St. Louis City Hospitals, he took up his old teaching job again at Washington University School of Medicine. With these and several other hospitals, he was associated for many years. At the university, he was Professor of Clinical Surgery from 1927 to 1941 and Professor Emeritus until his death. He was also appointed Professor of Oral Surgery at Washington University School of Dentistry from 1927 to 1941 and thereafter Professor Emeritus until he died.

His book *Surgery and Diseases of the Mouth and Jaws* was published in 1912, and it speedily became recognised as a classic, just as he too was soon to be recognised as an authority. The Surgeon General chose him to head the section of Oral and Plastic Surgery in the US Army, and he also became Chief Consultant in maxillofacial surgery with the American Expeditionary Forces during the First World War, when he spent 9 months in France and England.

It was at this stage of his career that he met Sir Harold Gillies. Gillies, perhaps, was more of an eccentric, but Blair too had his little ways, such as persisting in wearing old tennis shoes and gauze wound around his face and head in the theatre. Blair was keen on horsehair sutures, and it was said that he kept an old white horse at the Mullanphy Hospital so that whenever he needed a new supply of suture material, a few hairs could be pulled from the horse's tail and expeditiously sterilised. One of Blair's sons, an orthopaedic surgeon, believes this to be untrue. His operating room was profusely decorated with charming figures from nursery rhymes which he hoped would amuse both his little and older patients.

Both Blair and Gillies realise the enormous benefits which would accrue from the judicious use of combined dental and surgical expertise for cases of severe facial injury. Although Blair was well versed in anatomy of the jaws and had considerable experience in the treatment of jaw injuries, he had the very great good fortune to team up with Robert Ivy who possessed a qualification in dentistry as well as medicine. Ivy had been practising both maxillofacial and plastic surgery, and when he and Blair returned to America, they organised several army centres for the treatment of jaw and facial injuries.

There is no doubt that Blair was fast becoming the leading figure in the field of maxillofacial surgery in America, although he still considered himself a general surgeon. But from the 1920s onwards, he devoted himself almost entirely to plastic surgery, and his assistants were likewise trained mostly in plastic surgery. Earl Padgett, of dermatome fame, was the first on a list of men such as Canon, Barrett Brown (who later succeeded Blair as head of the department), Louis Byars and Frank McDowell, who were all later to become renowned in their specialty.

Besides his regular assistants, visitors from all over America came to learn the principles and observe the art of the developing specialty which Blair practised with skill and authority. From his writings, it can readily be seen that Blair's main interest was in head and neck surgery as well as the treatment of trauma and tumours of the jaws. Nowadays much of his early work would fall to the lot of the oral surgeon. Cleft lip and palate surgery was of great importance to him, and he was a strong opponent of traumatic procedures such as the wiring together of jaw elements as practised by Brophy. Incidentally, Brophy's own son-in-law, William Logan, who is now largely remembered for the Logan bow, was also against these rough techniques and, after careful study on infant cadavers, concluded that palatal closure with wiring was quite unsatisfactory.

In time, Blair's modification of the Mirault cleft lip operation became widely accepted in America, and although he discouraged people from attaching his name to the operation, he was not altogether successful in this respect. This exemplified his modesty, so often the hallmark of a great man, as did his refusal to accept the honour of becoming Chairman of The American Board of Plastic Surgery.

One of his most valuable contributions, together with James Barrett Brown, was the championing of large split skin grafts in place of the popular pinch and postage stamp grafts for burns and large granulating surfaces. Not only was the healing hastened by this technique but the end results were both cosmetically and functionally improved, thanks to a diminution in infection and the reduction of scar tissue. The skin grafting knife which he designed is not a museum piece, but in its day, this knife was far superior to the cut-throat razor which was widely used for removing small skin grafts. Blair also experimented with various devices to facilitate the taking of skin grafts, and eventually together with an instrument maker, he produced a suction box which drew the skin up in front on the knife and enabled grafts to be cut from the abdomen and chest.

The American Society of Plastic Surgeons was established in 1931 and has grown until today with 7,000 members. They are now surgeons who are certified by the American Board of Plastic Surgery which was the brainchild of Blair. In the 1930s, he became concerned with the growing impression in many quarters that plastic surgeons were nothing more than face lifters and nose whittlers. In order to rectify this misconception, he began to work for the acceptance of plastic surgery as a recognised specialty. By early 1937, he felt that his ideas had crystallised sufficiently to invite representatives from all over the country to discuss the establishment of a Plastic Surgery Board. The first meeting of the embryonic board took place on 14 June 1937, and although declining the chairmanship, Blair agreed to act as secretary. One of the main objects of the newly formed organisation was to lay down standards for the training and education of specialists, leading ultimately to their proper certification.

At his own expense, Blair travelled around America promulgating these ideas and getting to know the men who were to become members of the founding group. By degrees and much hard work, the many problems were solved, and although initially the Board was an affiliate of the American Board of Surgery, it was granted independent status in May 1941. The requirements laid down in those days have been steadily improved. Today the high standards continue to bear fruit in the expansion of this specialty and the valuable scientific contributions and their clinical applications, which flow from all over America.

The list of Blair's writings, which span more than half a century, is truly formidable. His three classic books, *Surgery and Diseases of the Mouth and Jaws*, *Essentials of Oral Surgery* and *Cancer of the Face and Mouth*, reflect his main field of endeavour, but he published almost 200 articles on a host of subjects varying from the care of premature infants to the treatment of burns. It is said that he had a flair for invention but, at the same time, appreciated the importance of basic science and its application to clinical practice, as evidenced by his work on wound healing. His literary style is widely revered in America and he was not above introducing a little whimsical honour to his scientific writings. Clearly, Blair possessed enormous energy, which found its outlet mainly in his work.

Blair was a soft-spoken, lanky man, with a slight stoop and silvery hair. He enjoyed a happy family life with his wife, three daughters and two sons and was a devout Catholic. Every summer, he sent his wife and children to their lakeside house in Wisconsin to get away from the oppressive heat of St. Louis. As he was very much involved with the treatment of children with clefts coming from all over America and wanted to be operated on in the summer holidays, he spent most of the summer with his nose to the grindstone.

Just outside St. Louis above the Missouri River, he bought an old house with about 13 acres of land called River View Farm where he enjoyed planning, building and renovating the buildings. It was here that he spent his declining years. Besides his work and family, he had few interests and his main hobby was collecting Oriental carpets. He even attempted to make his own miniature rugs using the proper knotting techniques which perhaps came easily to a surgeon.

He was especially devoted to his wife who had been born with a dislocated hip, but nevertheless she led an active life until struck down by a stroke in 1942. This illness was a terrible blow to Blair who devoted more and more time to the care of his wife. A bus was converted to a mobile home cum hospital, with additional sleeping accommodation for two nurses and a lift fixed to the bus so that his wife's wheelchair could be hoisted on board. This enabled Blair to travel in comfort with his wife and to spend holidays in various States and Canada.

Of the many honours that came his way, honorary membership of both British and American Associations of Plastic Surgeons, as well as the American Society of Plastic and Reconstructive Surgery, was perhaps the most important. He was a member or fellow of innumerable American Societies, and the list reflects his eclectic medical interests as well as the esteem in which this great pioneer in plastic surgery was held during his lifetime.

Chapter 12
John Staige Davis (1872–1946)

The First Real Plastic Surgeon

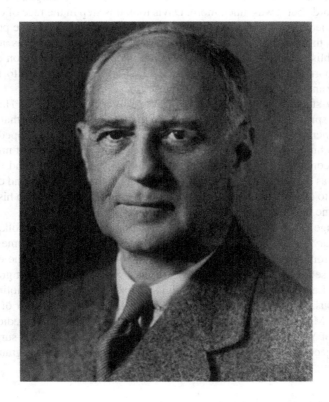

Understandably, doubt and dispute often surround claims to priority, a situation which is not unknown in the field of plastic surgery. There is good evidence to support my claim that Staige Davis was the first to declare that he was a full-time practising plastic surgeon and to suit his actions to his words. Although articles on his life and work do not make it entirely clear when he limited his surgical

© Springer International Publishing Switzerland 2015   45
D. Tolhurst, *Pioneers in Plastic Surgery*, DOI 10.1007/978-3-319-19539-1_12

endeavours to plastic surgery, his son, Dr. William Bowdoin Davis, told me that it was in 1909 that Staige Davis decided to practise only plastic surgery. Later, when going through family papers, I discovered that Staige Davis, himself, had written a very short summary of his life in which he says:

> In 1909, I limited my practice to plastic surgery
> and am Plastic Surgeon to several hospitals here.....!

It is true that Zeis coined the title *Plastische Chirurgie* in 1838 and that the names of a number of nineteenth- and early twentieth-century continental general and ENT surgeons such as Dieffenbach, von Graefe and Morestin are associated with a variety of reconstructive and cosmetic techniques but not one dared to name themselves plastic surgeons or saw the need for or dared to practise full-time plastic surgery. This visionary and bold first step belonged to Staige Davis.

Some may argue that the epithet of the 'First Real Plastic Surgeon' is simply a matter of words but it was much more. Davis took this step in the face of opposition which included that of the powerful Stewart Halsted and in due course proved that a practice in the specialty was viable. In addition, he showed that it was now necessary to establish proper training and research in the field. This was soon confirmed by the support and respect of his colleagues who joined with him to found the Association and the Board of Plastic Surgery.

To many students of the history of plastic surgery, the name of Harold Delf Gillies will spring to mind as the founder of the speciality. It is true that he, more than any other, except perhaps Johannes Esser, a Dutchman, developed and laid down the techniques and principles which even today form the basis of much of the plastic surgeon's work. Gillies, however, was initially an ear, nose and throat surgeon who was drawn to reconstructive surgery during the Great War, and only when he returned to civilian practice in 1919, 10 years after Davis had set up his practice, did he confine his practice solely to plastic surgery.

John Staige Davis was born a seventh-generation American in Norfolk, Virginia, on 15 January 1872. The family, whose lineage is quite well documented, was descended from Andrew Davis, who emigrated from Wales early in the eighteenth century and settled in Middlesex County, Virginia. Staige Davis's great grandfather, Professor of Law at the University of Virginia, was shot and killed by a rioting student on the campus. He left a son, John Staige Davis, who became Professor of Anatomy and Materia Medica. His son, William Blackford Davis, also studied medicine at the University of Virginia and became a naval and subsequently an army surgeon. His son, the subject of this account, was an only child and named after his grandfather.

Childhood and Student Life

As a young child, Staige Davis led a somewhat nomadic life, as his father's naval posting took the family in turn from Virginia to Maryland, Washington D.C. and New Hampshire. In 1877, his father was commissioned in the United States army, and it is from this period that young Staige Davis began to recall his adventurous childhood. With his father once more on the move, the family entrained at St. Louis bound for Bismarck and Jamestown in Dakota Territory. Upon arrival, they travelled in an ambulance, escorted by troops of the 7th Cavalry, through Indian country for 100 miles to Fort Totten. Although, by this time, the Indian wars had ended, the nearby Sioux were occasionally unfriendly, and Staige Davis could remember witnessing a skirmish between a squad of cavalry and two Indians who had murdered some settlers. Here, his father bought him a beautiful black mare from a friendly full-blooded Sioux.

The growing boy spent a fascinating time riding, visiting Sioux camps, tending the soldiers' horses, learning to drive mule wagons and hunting with his father during the next 8 years. One of his unpleasant memories was sampling some cigars with a friend, an experience which accounted for his lifelong aversion to tobacco!

Up until the age of 13, his parents had been responsible for his education, as there were few children and no school at the Fort. In 1885, he returned to the East Coast and spent 2 years at the Heathcote School in Buffalo and then in 1897 enrolled at the Episcopal High School of Virginia, where his uncle was the headmaster. This fortuitous family relationship and his father's adherence to the Episcopalian Church were no doubt factors influencing the choice of school. It was a Spartan existence with no heating nor running water, which prepared him for his next scholastic adventure at St. Paul's School in Garden City, Long Island, when his father was once again transferred, this time to New York. The pupils were here subjected to strict military discipline as well as a rigorous exposure to religion, with twice-daily chapel services and two cathedral parades in full dress uniform every Sunday.

He was released from this bondage upon graduation and passed on to Yale University at New Haven in 1892 where he did extremely well, making Phi Beta Kappa in his final year. Besides being invited to join the Book and Snake Society, he was captain of the Sheffield Military Company and elected to the Board of Editors of the Yale Scientific Monthly, which was founded by his class of 1895.

Entrance to a medical school in those days was not so fiercely contested as it is today, and Staige Davis debated between Harvard and Johns Hopkins Medical School. Oddly enough, the author had the same choice as a postgraduate fellow but, unlike Staige Davis, decided on Harvard in 1963. Seven of his companions from the Yale biology course accompanied him to Johns Hopkins where he and Paul Owsley decided to room together in Baltimore. For the first 2 years, they lived in a downtown boarding house and for the last two in an apartment on North Charles Street.

The medical faculty during the 4-year course boasted some of the most famous names in medicine. There were Welsh the pathologist, Kelly in gynaecology and, most notable of all, Osler, who favoured bedside teaching and provided a wonderful course, being in close contact with the third and fourth year medical students. Halsted, on the other hand, although one of the greatest of American general surgeons, was not interested in students whom, it was said, he barely tolerated. Furthermore, the great man contrived to restrict the teaching and development of subspecialties, such as orthopaedics, urology and ophthalmology, none of which interested him – a situation which is not altogether unknown to the author!

On the day of his graduation in 1899, Davis learned that he was amongst the top 12 in his class. It was the custom for this fortunate group to be offered a 12-month rotation at Hopkins as house officers, spread between such giants as Osler, Kelly and Williams in gynaecology and obstetrics and, of course, Halsted. Even though the first 4 months were spent on a ward full of 35 cases of typhoid fever, the young intern later wrote that this year had been a truly memorable experience.

Surgical Career

At the end of his internship, Staige Davis began a 3-year surgical residency at the Union Protestant Infirmary in Baltimore, later the Union Memorial Hospital, where, in time, he became a member of the visiting staff. In 1903, he opened an office as a general surgeon in Baltimore and became associated with the surgical dispensary at the Johns Hopkins and the Robert Garrett Hospital for Children. Two years later, he accepted a professorship at the Women's Medical College in Baltimore, a post which he resigned in 1908. During the years between 1909 and 1917, he spent much of his spare time in the Hunterian Laboratory of Experimental Surgery and engaged in research which later was to be the basis of some of his scientific papers. In addition, he was the resident physician at the Avalon Inn and the Chattolanee Hotel in the Greenspring Valley near Baltimore during the summer for 4 or 5 years before his marriage in 1907.

It was in about 1901 that Staige Davis began to develop an interest in plastic surgery. At this time, there were many general surgeons, in the true sense of the word, employing plastic surgical procedures as required. There were no full-time plastic surgeons or books in English on the subject, and very little, if any, instruction was given on the techniques in use. German surgery was then in its heyday, and as Davis himself said, even Halsted spent most of the time at his teaching clinics holding forth on the latest activities of his German colleagues.

Up until the turn of the century, names such as von Graefe, Dieffenbach and von Langenbeck virtually dominated the literary field of reconstructive surgery. These three, incidentally, were all predecessors of Professor von Bergman at the Second Surgical Clinic of Berlin where Erich Lexer trained in general surgery. True, there were sporadic accounts published in English on a variety of plastic surgical procedures, but they were few and far between. If one looks in early textbooks on plastic surgery, there is scarcely one English name in the chapter references relating to the nineteenth century. Davis' first paper describing the correction of a burn scar with a 'whole thickness' skin graft was published in 1907. More than 70 publications were to follow, including his book on plastic surgery published in 1919 and a chapter in Lewis's textbook *Practice of Surgery*.

By his own account, Davis limited his practice to plastic surgery from 1909 onwards. This may perhaps have differed somewhat from today's idea of what constituted the work of a plastic surgeon. But, if the contents of Staige Davis' book are anything to go by, there seems to be a close similarity between the causes and types of the many problems which we now treat, and on which he wrote. Not all would agree with the treatment he outlined, but more than 100 years have passed since his book appeared, and it is only natural that experience and research should have resulted in improvement. The wonder is that it has not been so dramatic!

One presumes that at first, Davis was not run off his feet, even though he had appointments at several hospitals, including Johns Hopkins. General surgeons died hard. A good deal of his time was spent in the laboratory between 1909 and 1917, no doubt whilst his name and reputation gathered momentum.

His father had not been wealthy, and even though he was an only child, Staige Davis had always experienced 'economy at home'. His allowance at the university was adequate but taught him to be careful with money, and this as he said 'kept me out of mischief!' According to one of his children, Staige Davis was comfortably off once settled in his private and married life.

America was late to enter the First World War, so that it was only in the summer of 1917 that the US Army began to realise that there was a need for surgeons with knowledge of plastic surgery. In a letter to Halsted, the Surgeon General's Office suggested that Staige Davis organise a course at Johns Hopkins for a selected group of surgeons, but Halsted scotched the idea. Moreover, Halsted actively discouraged Davis to succumb to the blandishments of several medical publishers, who, in 1917, proposed that he write a book on plastic surgery. In Halsted's mind, there was no need for such a work, and he advised Davis not to embark on the project as there would be no use for the book. Nevertheless, Davis decided to proceed with the book which was well illustrated with photographs and drawings made by his wife. It was published in 1919, and although he sent complimentary copies to a number of colleagues, only Halsted, Williams and Welsh reputedly failed to acknowledge Davis' kind gesture. Such boorish behaviour in three eminent medical figures must be attributed in some degree to professional jealousy or fear. On this note, one should reiterate that Halsted's antipathy towards the development of surgical specialities was no secret. The dampening effect of this attitude must have been very difficult and depressing, but Davis somehow found strength to continue with his dedication to plastic surgery in his conviction of its value to mankind.

During all his years as a visiting surgeon at Johns Hopkins, Davis never had any beds of his own. Even when Lewis succeeded Halsted, Davis continued in the outpatient dispensary but could hardly find enough inpatients to operate on, so that teaching of his residents was difficult. At length, Blalock, who followed Lewis as the Chief of Surgery, showed some appreciation by asking Davis, who, by 1942, had reached the age of 70, to stay on as Head of the Division of Plastic Surgery. But it was only when Longmire took over from Davis in 1943 that the plastic surgical service was immediately given 15 beds. Such was Staige Davis' reward for 43 years of faithful service to his alma mater! As I reflect on my days spent in the oldest university of the Netherlands, where I was lured by promises that never materialised, the reader may begin to understand my fascination and sympathy for this gentlemanly pioneer.

As if the difficulties at Hopkins were not enough (or perhaps because of them), Davis had for some time been troubled with worsening asthma. The specialists from whom he sought help attributed his problem to sinusitis and chronically infected tonsils and adenoids. They could do nothing for him. It was because of this ill-health that his attempt to join the Hopkins Unit in France in 1919 was unsuccessful. In the spring of 1920, he closed his office and moved with his family to the clean, dry air of Colorado. There, he was treated by an internist, and he also underwent several sinus operations over the ensuing 18 months. His wife, who had some money of her own, made this possible, as he did not work at all until he was pronounced cured.

The family returned to Baltimore and settled in the city. Davis opened a new office in Cathedral Street and began work in the mornings and rested in the afternoons. He re-established himself in the Union Memorial Hospital, and it was here that his teaching clinics began to attract the interest of colleagues. He also operated at Union Memorial Hospital, where he was assisted by young surgeons, amongst whom were Kitlowski, Neil Owens and his own son Bowdoin.

Clinical and Scientific Work

Now almost 50 and with more than 10 years of experience in plastic surgery, 30 odd scientific papers and his large book *Plastic Surgery: its Principles and Practice* behind him, Davis still faced an uphill struggle at Johns Hopkins. His practice in the city, however, began to flourish, and quite soon, he was acknowledged as the doyen of plastic surgery in his country. In 1925, his old university, Yale, conferred an Honorary Degree of Master of Arts on Davis, and the citation summarises his achievements most admirably: 'He has been a pioneer in plastic surgery. His voluminous treatise on the subject published in 1919 is an acknowledged authority. In this field, he stands at the head of his profession; he combined original research with practical services to humanity, stimulating the minds of his pupils and colleagues, and healing the bodies of sufferers'.

His papers cover a wide range and together with his book encompassed the entire scope of plastic surgery taught at that time. He was very fond of Z pasties, an advocate of skin grafts to speed the healing of wounds, wrote on his experience with bone and cartilage grafts and classified the different deformities found in cleft lip and palate patients.

The laboratory research, which was mostly carried out between 1909 and 1917, included such diverse subjects as haemangioma, pressure dressings, splinting of skin grafts and effects of scarlet red on the re-epithelialisation of skin graft donor sites. Some of his work was presented at meetings of the American Surgical Association and the Southern Surgical Association.

In the operating room, it seems he was not altogether at ease. He spoke little and then only of matters relating to the work on hand. He had a pronounced and unfortunate tremor and sweated profusely. To overcome his discomfort, he wore a piece of gauze over his forehead and under his cap as a sweat band. When he was recovering from his asthma, he used a metal mask rimmed with inflatable rubber, which was connected to a filter and outlet valve on his back, as he was afraid of the ether-saturated air expired by the patients. This apparatus was discarded in favour of two gauze masks when his fears proved unfounded.

During his operations, Staige Davis concentrated intensely and, despite his tremor, was a delicate, unhurried and meticulous surgeon. There were, as Pickrell says, 'never any verbal explosions.... even when things did not progress smoothly, but on these occasions, his tremor was more marked'. Like Gillies, if flaps or Z plastics did not fit well, Davis would patiently remove all the sutures, extend the incisions or undermine the skin, even several times if necessary, until he was satisfied, adding 'I believe this is better'. This was one of his rare flights into the realm of operating room conversation. Catgut was used for the subcutaneous tissue and fine silk or horse hair sutures for the skin. His assistants never carried out an operation themselves, even under supervision, but were on occasion allowed to insert the skin sutures.

As a clinician, he was absolutely honest, kind and reassuring to his patients and courteous to his colleagues and the nursing staff, in short, a true gentleman. The patients' social and financial status (if there is any difference) was apparently of no interest to him, certainly in so far as it affected the treatment, and his faithful secretary, Jessie Smith, and assistants were more attentive to the billing of private patients than Davis.

In time, surgeons from all over America and abroad came to visit him just as he himself had travelled widely to observe and study surgical techniques. He was at his best with small groups and uneasy and nervous when obliged to address a large assembly. Those who came found his patient and stimulating teaching sessions in the somewhat insalubrious atmosphere of the staff changing room, following operations to be most rewarding.

The American Board of Plastic Surgery was founded by a group of leading surgeons in 1937, and Davis was chosen as the first Chairman, an office he held from 1938 until his retirement in 1945. Amongst his many activities as an advisor or committee man was his membership of the Maryland Medical Preparedness Committee in 1940, Advisor to the Division of Medical Sciences of the National Research Council, Advisor to the Surgeon General, Chairman of the Council of the Southern Surgical Association, Regent of the American College of Surgeons (of which he was a founder member) and finally, in 1946, President of the American Association of Plastic Surgeons.

Home and Family Life

As a bachelor, in his early 30s, Staige Davis was handsome and easy-going. His winning manners and charm made him a popular figure in Baltimore society, where he was much in demand. Amongst his close friends, he was known as Sunshine, a name chosen because of his fun-loving nature and good sense of humour.

Prior to his 2-year engagement to Kathleen Bowdoin, he had dated her sister, Marion, 4 years her junior. Staige was 10 years older than Kathleen. The protracted engagement was attributed to a lack of money, and by the time he felt secure enough to tie the matrimonial knot, Davis had been in surgical practice for about 5 years. After a honeymoon in the Adirondacks, the newlyweds settled in Baltimore and were blessed by the birth of three children: Kathleen (now Kay Darlington) was the oldest, and William Bowdoin and Howland were the two sons. Bowdoin later took up plastic surgery and Howland became a pilot.

Whilst the children were young, the couple kept two nursemaids so Staige Davis' prudent preparation for marriage enabled the family to live in considerable comfort. The only concern in these early years was a persistent tendency to upper respiratory infections to which he attributed the development of asthma. As it will be remembered, Davis was obliged to close his practice and move out to Colorado Springs because of his illness. Here, intensive treatment over the course of 18 months helped him overcome his problems.

Upon his return to Baltimore in 1921, Davis built a comfortable house at 215 Wendover Road on a plot next door to his wife's sister, now Marion Knox. There he soon established an excellent ménage, sporting five servants, including a cook, a maid, a laundress, Steward the gardener/chauffeur and James the butler. The family led a quiet, conventional life, rubbing shoulders with members of the old established Baltimore families but not competing in the lists of high society. He had two or three close friends, but in his free time, life centred round his family.

The daily routine began reasonably early, as Davis preferred to begin operating at 8 o'clock. He was not a compulsive late worker like some surgeons who never seem able to finish a day's work in the space of 12 to 14 hours. As a rule, he was home in time to enjoy dinner with the family. In the evening, he passed the time reading or listening to music rather than going out to his clubs and retired to bed about 10 o'clock. Davis was an avid reader of biographies and spy, detective and western novels. As a young man, he had flirted with the guitar, but in later life, he confined his musical efforts to light-hearted whistling!

On Sundays, his wife was rarely able to convince him of the wisdom of accompanying her to church; whilst she was very fond of and active in the church, her husband's religion in a sense was his work. He usually held an outpatient clinic at the Union Memorial Hospital on Sunday mornings for people who found it difficult to travel to the hospital or miss their work during the week. There was always a large family breakfast on Sundays and a lunch following the clinic to which interns or out-of-town staff were invited.

The family led an orderly life. Summer vacations were spent in Maine or Fishers Island off the coast of Connecticut – the family travels there by train. In the winter, they usually took 3 weeks in Florida. Robert Miller, a friend of Davis' and a thoracic surgeon, and his family often accompanied them. During these breaks, Staige Davis was fond of riding, canoeing and swimming, but a swollen leg from thrombosis, the legacy of a ruptured appendix and scarlet fever at the same time, had obliged him to give up more active sports such as golf and tennis. He had no real card sense and was unsuccessful in attempting to master the intricacies of bridge.

Like most good Americans, he had a weakness for cars and over the years experimented with many different makes, usually changing them every 2 years. Ultimately, he settled on Buicks, like the author, who looks back fondly on his 1927 and 1956 models. Davis usually drove himself although Steward, the chauffeur and gardener, was with the family for almost 50 years. In his 60s, his wife persuaded her husband to surrender the controls to Steward, who drove Davis to and from the hospital each day. Prior to this arrangement, Davis had the services of Fred, a German immigrant and instrument maker, who also helped to look after the car.

Staige Davis was just over 6 feet tall with brown hair and eyes. His hair turned to silver-grey in his later years, and this added to his distinguished appearance. He was neat and clean, particular about his clothes, which were as conservative as the man who wore them, and he scarcely ever appeared without a tie, even when relaxing at the weekend. Every morning, he carefully wound an ace bandage around his swollen leg before choosing his shoes, which were always polished by James the butler, 'till they shone like mirrors'. He never smoked and only drank in moderation, usually when on holiday and never if he was on duty. His daughter was in her teens during the prohibition era, and her father was terrified she might be poisoned by bathtub gin, taken surreptitiously from a hip flask. At her coming-out party, there was only alcohol-free punch available to drink.

Both his daughter and son to whom I have spoken remembered him as a serious man where important issues were at stake. He was not austere and a twinkle in his eye hinted at a fine sense of humour. The children still comment on their father's engaging smile and his compassion and concern for all his patients. No one was ever refused treatment because they were unable to afford payment. Davis' faithful secretary, Jessie Smith, looked after the financial side of the practice, and her astute investments left him more comfortably off than he had expected when he finally retired in 1945. From then on, he lived quietly in the family house and died peacefully there on 23 December 1946. His wife died at the age of 93 on exactly the same day 30 years later.

Many young surgeons, in fact the vast majority of those to whom I have spoken, do not know who Staige Davis was, and scarcely anyone at all in Europe realises that he has the right to be dignified by the title of 'The First True Plastic Surgeon'. In his home town and at Johns Hopkins, he is accorded the distinction he deserves. The medical faculty founded the Staige Davis Society, and there is an archive at the Children's Hospital in Baltimore, where a collection of Davis' papers and writings, as well as some photographs and instruments, are preserved for all who are interested in the work of this true forefather of the profession of plastic surgery.

Chapter 13
Johannes Fredericus Samuel Esser (1877–1946)

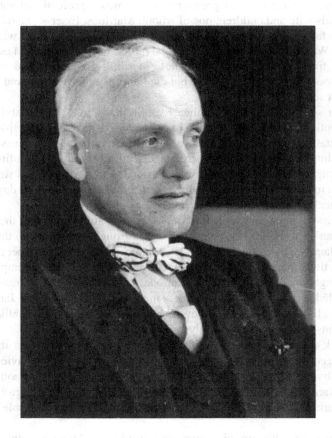

The specialty of plastic and reconstructive surgery was officially recognised in Holland in 1950, the same year in which Dr. C.F. Koch, the doyen and the first post-war specialist in this branch of surgery, founded on his own initiative the Dutch

© Springer International Publishing Switzerland 2015
D. Tolhurst, *Pioneers in Plastic Surgery*, DOI 10.1007/978-3-319-19539-1_13

Society of Plastic and Reconstructive Surgery. Charles Koch was already a busy general surgeon in Zeeland when the Wehrmacht invaded Holland, but he attached himself to a French battalion and managed to escape to England where he was persuaded by Archibald McIndoe to gain experience in plastic surgery. When Koch returned to Amsterdam after the Second World War, little was known in Holland of another Dutch pioneer in this branch of surgery, Johannes Esser, largely because he had spent most of his working life outside his native country.

In 1946, Johannes Fredericus Samuel Esser died a lonely death in Chicago, after a remarkable and fascinating life, highlighted by the development of many original principles and operation techniques in plastic surgery. Beyond the borders of his native country, he had enjoyed an international reputation for 30 years yet even now his name is not as well known as it deserves to be.

Jan Esser was descended from an old military family who came from the Dutch university town of Leiden. His great-grandfather was a professional soldier who abandoned his wife and children, one of whom, Martinus, Esser's grandfather, followed in his father's footsteps. Revolted by the bloody battle scenes he witnessed in the Belgian War of Independence in 1831, he retired to civilian life and established one of the first life insurance companies. Martinus Esser had two sons. One embarked upon the study of medicine but died during a dreadful typhoid epidemic whilst still a student.

His other son was Jan Esser's father. Even in those times, his lifestyle was far from conventional. He was not in the least interested in study and rapidly abandoned a flirtation with the law in order to pursue his principle interests amongst many of riding, music and art. His marriage with a ravishingly beautiful girl of French Huguenot descent who sold strawberries led to a rift with his strict father who refused to meet the girl or her family. Such a mesalliance in those days was no trifling matter!

In 1877, a son, Jan, was born to the couple one year after the birth of their daughter, Betsy. Jan's upbringing was complicated and strongly influenced by three members of the family. His mother attended to religious instruction, his father to general knowledge, the appreciation of art and music and his grandfather attempted to set him on the right toad by imparting conventional wisdom to the young man. A sound basic knowledge of economy and business matters were instilled into Jan Esser at an early age, but his broad general development on the home front conflicted with school lessons, which he pursued only under duress.

An attack of acute rheumatism in his youth wrongly was at first thought to have damaged his health. He was sorely plagued by the odd behaviour of his father who lived in a workers' quarter of the city where he attracted considerable adverse criticism by such eccentricities as leading his horse through his house over the marble floors, as this was the only manner whereby the stable could be reached.

When Esser was thirteen, his father died of a heart ailment, and this loss was speedily followed by that of his grandfather. His mother became introspective and depressive, and as she became more and more of a recluse, she was unable to care for her children.

Although still in his teens, the young Esser was already independent enough to successfully negotiate the sale of the family home and the purchase of a new property. This was the beginning of the considerable acumen he was to demonstrate in the business world. The budding businessman's talents were far reaching for he soon distinguished himself as a chess player and in quick order defeated all the renowned players in Leiden. Together with a group of fellow students from the lyceum, he formed a new club, which rapidly achieved national recognition.

Deterioration in his mother's health led to her being admitted to a hospital, and her children were then placed with foster families. Their normal schooling continued and in Esser's case so successfully that he gained a place at Leiden, the oldest University in Holland to study medicine. Early on he developed a profound interest in anatomy which led to his assembling a remarkable collection of malformed skulls. However, he maintained his interest in chess, often playing in tournaments abroad, and wrote a column for a daily paper, which paid enough for him to complete his medical studies in comfort. During this period, he helped his sister, who had enrolled at the dental school, with her studies, but he was such a demanding taskmaster; she often dissolved into tears during her brother's tutorials! Such was his industry that Esser also attended lectures at the dental school and somehow managed to complete the theoretical part of the course during his medical studies. He and his sister then moved to Utrecht where the practical course was given.

In 1903, he graduated in medicine from the University of Leiden and shortly thereafter was crowned Dutch National Chess Champion. For a brief period, he worked as a locum tenens in general practices in Holland before completing his doctoral thesis at Gent in an amazingly short time. He then set sail for South America as ship's surgeon and during the voyage visited both Central and North America. The captain in whom Esser found a worthy chess opponent telegraphed ahead to the chess fraternity in Caracas that the Dutch champion was on board and a tournament was organised in which Esser took part on his arrival.

Upon his return to Holland in 1904, he set up in practice as a country doctor in the tiny, remote village of Polsbroek. There he purchased a noisy motorbike in order to get around his practice and also acquired two Irish Setters, which found the chickens in the neighbourhood splendid sport. The villagers disapproved of their new doctor's lifestyle, but the discontent was mutual, and after eighteen months, he exchanged his practice for one in Amsterdam where once again he was able to enjoy chess and his cultural interests. Back in the city, he organised a new chess club (which is still in existence), and his house soon became a centre for art lovers for whom he organised exhibitions and art evenings. A new storey was added to his house to accommodate these activities. Paintings and antique furniture filled his home, and soon his time was equally divided between his practice and his love of art.

Amongst his many friends in the art world were Breitner, Witsen, Mondriaan and Sluijters, most of whom were still unknown. True to form, Esser's appreciation of his art collection did not exclude its financial value, and he assembled hundreds of paintings with an eye to the future. He never came away empty-handed from the studios of his friends and even took with him canvasses they had consigned to the rubbish bin. When some of these resurrected works were later exhibited by Esser, Breitner, amongst others, expressed his extreme displeasure, and the two fell out.

In 1912 at the age of thirty-five, Esser met Olga Hazelhoff-Roelfzema, whom he quickly married, and the two set off on their honeymoon by train for Russia, which in those days was considered almost at the other end of the world!

Then, just as his life and practice in a smart area of Amsterdam began to blossom, Esser decided to throw everything up for a career that he thought would better suit his talents. He had always harboured a considerable interest in the face and its congenital malformations as well as abnormalities caused by accident or disease, so the family moved to Utrecht where Esser embarked on the study of general surgery under Professor Lameris. The training seemed unnecessarily lengthy and arduous to Esser so after one year he took his wife and daughter to Paris, where Professor Sebileau held courses for French military surgeons. Once over, he worked for six months with Hippolyte Morestin, the man who had influenced Gillies, and thereafter spent four months with Tuffier. In those days in France, as opposed to Holland, there was no problem in obtaining cadavers for dissection, and Esser made good use of this facility by working out many of the principles and techniques which he would later use as a plastic surgeon.

When the First World War broke out in 1914, he offered his services to the French and English governments, but both refused him on the grounds that he was a foreigner! Disappointed, he decided to return to Holland which was still neutral. In 1915, he began to work with Noordenbos in Rotterdam at the Bergweg Hospital and also at the Coolsingel Hospital, the forerunner of Rotterdam's University Hospital, where he concentrated on plastic surgery procedures. When he offered his services for the care of the wounded for the third time, it was to the Austro-Hungarian government, which was delighted to accept Esser on the condition he brought his own team with him. As soon as he heard the news, he departed for Czechoslovakia taking four operating theatre sisters, including the head sister, no doubt to the annoyance of his chief Noordenbos. For the first eight months until the beginning of 1916, he was busy in the enormous 3,600-bed military hospital at Brunn (now Brno) in Czechoslovakia, where he speedily began to make a considerable name for himself. He operated on a large number of cases and gave lectures, and a whole series of papers began to flow from his pen.

His fame quickly spread to Vienna to which he was invited to perform an operation at the University Clinic of Professor Julius von Hochenegg. The patient who suffered from an absence of the lower lip was one upon whom Hochenegg himself had operated several times. Before a full lecture theatre, the famous young Dutchman and his own theatre sister corrected the deformity with bilateral nasolabial flaps in one procedure, whilst Hochenegg gave a running commentary. Such was the success of this appearance that orders were issued that all wounded soldiers needing plastic surgery were to be sent to Esser. In January 1916, he moved to the University Clinic in Vienna, but after eight months, he was off again, this time to Budapest where he found the working conditions under Professor Onodi and Verebely more to his liking. There Mrs. Esser, even though she had no training, assisted her husband with his operations, whilst their daughter played between the barracks amongst patients whose faces were in various stages of reconstruction.

Publications of his results, richly illustrated with pre- and postoperative photographs, continued to appear in German and American journals. Through the latter, his work came to the attention of Gillies and his colleagues at Sidcup, who spoke of the Esser-inlay as 'marking an epoch in surgery'. This technique was modified by Waldron and Gillies who called it the 'Esser-outlay', and this idea then crossed the Atlantic thanks to propaganda from Gillies and his returning American students. All this while Esser's work remained virtually unheard of in his own native neutral Holland!

Following a visit to Lexer, then a general surgeon in Jena, who was extremely interested in reconstructive surgery, Esser wrote to Professor Bier suggesting a plan for the establishment of a department for plastic surgery in Bier's clinic at the University of Berlin which involved cooperation with the departments of general surgery, ophthalmology and dentistry. Bier, Kruckmann and Schroder then invited Esser to Berlin and so began a remarkable and perhaps his most flourishing period as a reconstructive surgeon. His first book on cheek rotation flaps appeared in 1918 and immediately sold out. It was designed to outline the general principles of plastic surgery and aimed in particular at military surgeons. Although major wounds of the head and neck were commonplace in trench warfare, the standard of reconstruction was indifferent, and Esser's proposed methods were quite revolutionary.

In Berlin, Esser had a department with 150 beds at his disposal, but he also operated in several other clinics in the city as well as travelling throughout Germany to operate at many other centres. The value of his work was fully recognised, and he was accorded the title of Doctor in Germany without examination. Somewhat later, he became a lecturer at the Prussian Surgical Academy where in 1922 he held a course on reconstructive surgery. Maliniac, the founder of the American Society for Plastic Surgery, attended this course, and one of Esser's pupils in Berlin at this time, who later achieved world renown, was Gustave Aufricht. Esser's activities as a surgeon and organiser could almost be described as frenzied, and he had made such an impression in Germany that he was proposed as a professor at Berlin University. Due to the changing political atmosphere, the decline in the economy and also to the death of his young wife in 1923, his appointment at the last moment was not realised. Somehow Esser survived a miserable period of disappointment and depression which came at the end of nearly a decade spent mostly in Germany. Once again he returned to Amsterdam where he bought several houses and moved restlessly from one to another. It was there that the idea came to him of setting up an international centre for plastic surgery whose principal aims were to be the training of young surgeons and the treatment and rehabilitation of social outcasts.

He decided to settle in France but for the next three years led a peripatetic existence, operating almost exclusively by invitation on difficult cases all over France as well as in Belgium, England and Holland. His energy seemed to know no limits for upon receipt of a telegram in Amsterdam he would proceed by train to Paris and from there to London or Brussels. It was in London that he made the acquaintance of Sir Harold Gillies and other well-known specialists such as Eastman Sheehan.

With the purchase of a splendid castle in France in 1927 which was to be the site of his institute, it seemed as if his plans would come to fruition, but the French Government began to cause difficulties, apparently because he was a foreigner. As a solution to these problems, Esser turned to the idea of an extraterritorial centre, rather like the Red Cross, which would be answerable to the League of Nations, and he sought advice and assistance from Professor Faure and several international lawyers.

Typically, he found enough time to fit in an extensive voyage in 1928, during which he operated in South America. Many ex-convicts from Devil's Island, who had been mauled by sharks or whose faces were covered with obscene tattoos, attracted his interest, and he did much to try and reintegrate them in society.

In 1929, he remarried Aleida de Koning who had nursed him in Leiden when he was recovering from an appendectomy. She bore him three daughters. The family settled in Monaco where the tax and winter climates were to Esser's liking. Summers were spent in Esser's castle near Tours and the colder months in Monaco. Upon his return to France from South America, he approached the French Government and suggested it buy several small islands with the amusing names of Le Pere, La Mere, Les Mamelles and Malingre upon which he proposed to establish his centre, but his request was refused. However, Esser who had tasted disappointment before was not easily discouraged, and he launched an intensive campaign in Europe in which he concentrated on many important government representatives and heads of state in order to win them over to his cause. His humanitarian idealism brought him considerable support amongst eminent scientists and Nobel Prize winners who in turn attracted further interest in the project.

As a diplomat, he was not a success for he had no love of protocol, and attempts to influence leading statesmen were regarded as clumsy. The pompous Mussolini, for example, was not impressed by Esser, who had no interest or feeling for politics. This was unfortunate, as Esser needed the support of several fascist leaders for his dream of an independent island in the Mediterranean. In 1934, the official establishment in Paris of the 'Institut Esser de Chirurgie Structive' took place, but Esser continued his apostolic travels throughout Europe in the name of his institute where he foresaw the possibility of dealing with a waiting list which he estimated at four million cases, most of whom would require plastic surgery.

All this time, he was busy churning out articles and books, the royalties from which he imagined would help to finance his grandiose project. A short monograph on 'Ear Plastic' appeared in 1926, and this was followed by the first edition of perhaps his best work 'Artery Flaps' in 1929, which was reprinted in 1932.

At last in 1938, it seemed as if his goal was in sight for the King of Greece and leading intellectuals showed not only enthusiasm but active cooperation for his plans. A Greek torpedo boat, the Niki, was put at his disposal, and Esser cruised the Aegean Sea until he came upon the island of Kyra Panagia which seemed the ideal spot. These activities attracted interest from the press and articles began to appear in French and Dutch papers as well as weekly magazines and little wonder for there had been no project like this since the founding of the Red Cross. At this moment, when success was in sight, the Second World War broke out; Poland collapsed and all eyes were turned to Germany. Characteristically, Esser once more offered his services to France, but they were foolishly declined on the grounds that he had helped the Austro-Hungarians during the Great War.

Once again disappointed but not dispirited, Esser and his eldest son boarded a boat for America where they still hoped to find support for the dream of an international institute. However, in the United States, he was greeted with distrust, born of jealousy of his famous talents as an organiser. For the first twelve months, he lived in a state close to poverty, as he had brought no capital with him, for he had intended a relatively short stay, and the way back to Europe was soon cut off. The two men bought a Ford pickup and converted it into a camping wagon in which they crisscrossed America for a year. His son acted as chauffeur as Esser did not possess a driving license. In France, his attempts to master the mysteries of a large Panhard had resulted in an unfortunate accident! His ingenuity proved unequal to the task of controlling the car, which careered into the front of a greengrocer's shop leaving Esser shaken and disillusioned with this form of self transport.

Finally, in 1941, Esser managed to purchase a large dilapidated house in Chicago, which was repaired and renovated. He began to build up contacts, especially with university clinics, and although as a foreigner, he was strictly not permitted to operate in America, he was invited to do so because of his reputation. In the early 1940s, a severe Dupuytren's contracture put an end to his active surgical career, but he carried on lecturing and writing, devoting much of his time during this period to philosophy. By degrees, his heart began to fail and digitalisation proved of no help. In 1946, he collapsed in front of his house in Chicago and died at the age of 69.

Esser was a tall, slim man who held himself erect. He was good looking and clean-shaven with dark blond hair, which he wore in the crew cut style as a student. In America, he aged rapidly and became almost totally bald. He had no feeling for fashion and cared little for his clothes. During his many train trips, he was in the habit of travelling in two suits so that upon arrival he could throw off the topmost of the two, thereby saving time!

He left behind more than 150 publications, including several books and atlases on war injuries, which were translated into many languages as well as fantastic art and antique collections. Strangely enough, he never published a single article in the Dutch language. One year after his sad and lonely death, Holland's first plastic surgeon, Dr. Charles Koch, began his practice in Amsterdam.

Chapter 14
Frantisek Burian (1881–1965)

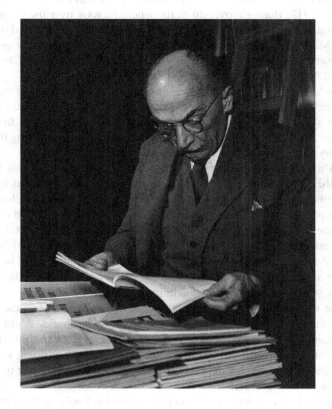

Those who knew him well say that Burian ranked with Gillies, Esser, Kilner and McIndoe as one of the masters and founders of modern plastic surgery. Burian was born in Prague on 17 September 1881, exactly 9 months to the day before Sir Harold Gillies was born. He studied medicine at Charles University in Prague, and

© Springer International Publishing Switzerland 2015

D. Tolhurst, *Pioneers in Plastic Surgery*, DOI 10.1007/978-3-319-19539-1_14

following his graduation, he spent 1 year at the Institute of Pathology before starting on his surgical training in 1907 at the First Department of Surgery.

At the outbreak of the Balkan Wars (1912–1913), Burian was working as surgical assistant to Professor Kukula in Prague, but he joined the surgical team of Professor Tobiasek in October 1912 and set out for Belgrade. The wars brought about a tremendous feeling of unity amongst the Slavs, and even those countries which were not directly involved in the conflict willingly came to the help of their neighbours. Professor Kukula had responded to the requests for help by the Bulgarian Red Cross and formed a medical team composed largely of Slavs from Prague, which was second in size only to that of the Russians.

The wars were of the old-fashioned type with open fighting, infantry attacks and cavalry encounters, which produced none of the dreadful destructive facial injuries seen in the First World War. Nevertheless, Burian became interested in facial wounds and made a study of the reconstructive possibilities, such as they were at this time.

In January 1913, Burian moved to Sofia, where he took over the second Czech Mission in the Military Hospital from Karel Stepan. The Mission settled on the first floor of the Military Academy in Sofia where Burian cleared the rooms and halls of all unnecessary furniture in order to reduce infection. He had 400 beds at his disposal, and he soon showed his colours as a good administrator.

The records, complete with sketches by Burian, are extant and reveal that besides his interest in facial wounds, he was heavily involved with all the skull and brain injuries. His wife, Anna Lakasora-Burianova, who was one of the very first women to graduate as a doctor under the Austrian monarchy, assisted him during this period and, for many years thereafter, was his only assistant.

One of Burian's earliest attempts at plastic surgery dates from this time. His notes describe a flap comprising the skin, muscle and bone, which was transposed from the forehead to correct a large defect in the face. It is said that he also began to use the tube pedicle before Gillies and Filatov, but in all modesty, he did not mention this matter when he gave the third Gillies Memorial Lecture in 1963.

With the advent of the First World War, Burian was appointed Chief Surgeon to the Eastern Austro-Hungarian Army in Temesvar in Romania. There, he began to devote more and more time to reconstructive surgery, not only of the face but also of the limbs, which led him to stress the importance of rehabilitation.

When the war ended, Burian gathered all his Czech patients together and had them transported back to Prague in a special train, in order that he could complete their treatment. This was an extremely difficult period, as he was obliged to move his department twice and his critics maintained that what he was doing was art, not science. However, he struggled on, and as his results began to speak for themselves, his ridiculous critics were silenced.

Gradually, he began to attract civilian patients and not only cases of trauma but children with facial, limb and genital deformities. Soon, he was asked to operate in children's institutions all over the country. The small department he had established in the Red Cross Hospital in 1921 grew until he was granted permission to move to the State Hospital in 1937, but he had to wait until 1948 before his department became part of the medical faculty in Prague.

Abounding with energy, fired by enthusiasm for his work and, furthermore, possessed of a dogged determination, he steadily overcame the obstructions which lay in his path, until he was appointed associate professor at Charles University in 1929, having twice been denied the post on the spurious ground that his work was not scientific. Apart from his surgical skill, his publications had attracted attention and he lectured and began to travel widely. His first notable book was entitled *Physiological Operating Techniques*, and this gives one an idea of the importance he attached to basic science and research.

Plastic surgery was accepted as a specialty at Charles University in 1929, and 3 years later, it was legally recognised in Czechoslovakia (the first country in the world to do so), which enabled Burian to employ permanent assistants. Both America and Great Britain may have acknowledged that plastic surgery was a blossoming specialty at this time, but it was only in 1941 that a Board of Plastic Surgery was granted independent status in the USA, thus paving the way for the proper training of assistants. It was not until 1946 that the British followed suit and established the Association of Plastic Surgeons.

Surgeons from his own country and abroad began to surround him, and he trained many foreigners who returned to establish the specialty of plastic surgery in their own lands. For example, he is still regarded as the founder of plastic surgery in Poland. Converse, who visited Burian in 1938, considered that he had the finest plastic surgery service and training programme in the world at that time. When the jackboots tramped into Prague in 1938, Burian's academic work was interrupted as the Nazis closed down the universities, and it was not until 1948 that Burian became a full professor and was granted his own department.

1954 and 1957 saw the publication of two additional books: *Surgery of Cheilopalatal Clefts* and *Rare Congenital Defects of the Face and Skull and their Treatment*. In 1956, a scientific research centre was set up. This was largely concerned with skin transplantation and congenital anomalies. Cleft lip and palate surgery particularly attracted him, and his technique for lip closure became known as the Prague method. Several operations have been dignified by Burian's name, and amongst the best known of his innovations are techniques for suspending the ptotic eyelid, correcting chordee in hypospadias, lining a newly made vagina with a full-thickness skin graft and contour remodelling of the facial bones with cartilage.

It was Burian who had the idea, organising ability and determination to establish a central registry for congenital deformities for the whole of Czechoslovakia, and later, he tried to coordinate research into these problems at an international level. He continued to write and lecture long after he retired from the university and, as he grew older, was often seen leaning on the arm of his delightful and devoted daughter, Olga, during his travels. In retirement, he stayed on as a director of the research centre which had by then been incorporated into the Czechoslovak Academy of Science.

Honoured many times in his own country for both his scientific and humanitarian contributions, he was universally popular abroad as both speaker and visitor. The British Association of Plastic Surgeons made him an honorary member, but he was also an active member of societies in France, Germany, Belgium, America and Argentina.

Professor Burian was a short man who, as he grew older, bore the double burden of a marked kyphosis and deafness with great courage and not without humour. He said that the advantage of a hearing aid was that one could turn it off during boring lectures and speeches. The mention of his name brings to mind a bow tie, steel-rimmed spectacles and a bristling white moustache, which bespoke a pugnacious spirit, when the situation so demanded.

Beyond the boundaries of his special technical, creative and scientific skills lay a zest for life embracing a love of nature and a talent for drawing and painting. He was very fond of hiking in the Giant Mountains near his beloved country cottage, where he also skied regularly right up until a few months before his death.

In the 1981 issue of Acta Chirurgiae Plasticae, dedicated to his memory, those who wrote about this great man spoke of his brilliant mind, his unfailing energy, courage and determination… who was a skilful surgeon, dedicated scientist and sympathetic teacher. However, above all and through his humanitarian warmth, he occupied a special place in the hearts of his many friends.

Chapter 15
Sir Harold Delf Gillies (1882–1960)

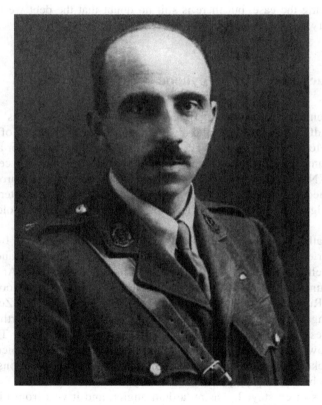

In 1918, as the rumble of the guns died away and peace spread over Europe once again, a new surgical seed, sown in the muddy battlefields of France, was growing slowly towards the light. Out of all the senseless slaughter, pain and grief of war came one good thing at least, and that was plastic surgery. In England, Gillies was

© Springer International Publishing Switzerland 2015
D. Tolhurst, *Pioneers in Plastic Surgery*, DOI 10.1007/978-3-319-19539-1_15

the man who nurtured and cultivated the growing specialty and in the post-war years had the courage to commit himself entirely to the practice of this new branch of surgery when others said it was impossible so to make a living. In the beginning, it was Gillies who trod his path alone, but in 1919, he was joined by Kilner, and in the early 1930s, two other New Zealanders, McIndoe and Mowlem, formed the quartet, which subsequently gave the impetus to the dissemination of the principles and possibilities of this new surgical specialty. By the outbreak of the Second World War, it was firmly rooted and has continued to grow in strength and stature.

Whatever is said about the infancy of plastic surgery, Sir Heneage Ogilvie probably best summed up the thoughts of the more perspicacious of Gillies' contemporaries when he wrote, 'Gillies invented plastic surgery. There was no plastic surgery before he came. Everything since then no matter whose name be attached to it was started by Gillies'. Now, 54 years after Gillies' death, one might say that Ogilvie was overstating the case, but there is still no doubt that the debt we owe to Sir Harold is very considerable indeed.

Family Background and Boyhood

For many generations, the Isle of Bute had been the home of Gillies' ancestors, but his grandfather, opposed to the disestablishment of the Church of Scotland, sailed away to New Zealand in 1852, where he qualified as a solicitor and subsequently became a magistrate in Dunedin, which for the best part of a century was the home of New Zealand's only medical school. His son Robert, Harold Gillies' father, married Emily Street, a great-niece of Edward Lear the painter, poet and humorist. Eight children were born to the couple, of whom Harold was the youngest.

Gillies' father was a successful land agent in Dunedin and sat for one session as a member of parliament. When he died in 1886, he left his wife and children relatively well provided for, and Emily Gillies moved to Auckland. At the tender age of 8, young Harold was taken by his mother to a preparatory school, Lindley Lodge near Rugby, in England. Four years later, he returned to New Zealand and entered Wanganui Collegiate School, also the alma mater of Sir Arthur Porritt, one-time president of the Royal College of Surgeons of England. The school boasted its own golf course, but Gillies was in those days preoccupied with the game of cricket, having become captain of the school eleven and considered by some as the best young player in the country. His brother, Bob, a farmer with whom Gillies often stayed, was an ardent angler, and it was from him that he acquired the rudiments of the art of fly fishing, at which he later so admirably excelled.

University and Hospital Days

Gillies followed two elder brothers to Cambridge University in England, where he had decided to study medicine. Law was the profession chosen by his brothers, but young Harold thought it desirable to expand the family horizons. His baritone voice won him a chapel scholarship, which was withdrawn when it was discovered that he had used the £40 for the purchase of a motorbike, and at this period, he left his mark more upon the sporting than the academic scene. He won a rowing Blue and a Half Blue for golf, at which he represented the university from 1903 to 1905 and whilst still up at varsity reached the semi-finals of the British Amateur Golf Championship.

In those days, Giles, as his friends called him, had already begun to make a name for himself as a practical joker, a foible which to some became an irritating and often exasperating quirk in later years. His habit of fixing his false teeth to walls with chewing gum, his ribald stories told in the then prudish society, a fondness for fanciful disguises, to say nothing of such eccentricities as wearing two neckties or a woman's hairnet or even make-up, can be ascribed to his dissatisfaction with meaningless convention as well as his zest for fun and life in general.

After Cambridge, he finished his medical studies at St. Bartholomew's Hospital in London, from which he graduated in 1908. By then, he had also shown a penchant for hard work and was highly thought of by the medical staff. He became a fellow of the Royal College of Surgeons in 1910. Following a period as house surgeon to D'Arcy Power at St. Bartholomew's Hospital, he began to climb the hierarchical ladder of ear, nose and throat surgery. In succession, he was chief assistant to Harmer at Barts, Registrar at the Hospital for Diseases of the Throat in Golden Square (of pump fame) and shortly after was appointed private assistant to Sir Milsom Rees.

Anxious to secure a foothold in the fashionable and lucrative sphere of private practice, which centred then, as it still does, on Wimpole and Harley Street, Gillies had hired morning dress for the interview with Rees. Sir Milsom evinced no interest in this sartorial spectacle or the candidate's qualifications, and Gillies' disappointment was further compounded when Sir Milsom produced his golf clubs for Gillies to inspect, since the great man was well aware of Gillies' golfing prowess. A discussion on the game and a demonstration by Sir Milsom of his own techniques were abruptly ended by the arrival of a patient. Almost as an afterthought, Sir Milsom exclaimed, 'Oh, my dear fellow; I'd forgotten.........the job. Well how would five hundred a year suit you?'

So, with this princely offer, began an association that lasted until 1915. Milsom Rees was an influential character, but his practice was rather unconventional, being principally devoted to the care of the voice. He listed among his appointments those of laryngologist to the King and Queen, as well as the royal household, and consultant to the Royal Opera House. It was there, whilst deputising for Sir Milsom, that the famous scissor accident occurred and Gillies was called to attend to a ballerina who had sat upon the offending instrument and 'injured a part of her body far removed from the larynx'.

With the improvement of his circumstances came marriage to the sister in charge of the new ENT department at Barts. Gillies, as a tolerable violinist, shared a love of music with his new wife, herself an accomplished pianist. Later in life, with their children, they played together as a quartet en famille. This happy marriage lasted until her death in 1957.

The First World War

When the war broke out, Gillies volunteered for the Red Cross, and in 1915, he was sent as a general surgeon to a Belgian ambulance in France. It was about this time that he met Charles Valadier, a flamboyant individual who had obtained a dental degree in Philadelphia. The stout, sandy-haired dentist had established a fashionable practice in Paris and was then touring about in his Rolls Royce, which Gillies said had been fitted out as a mobile dental office, attending to the teeth of the imperial general staff. He was able to convince the generals of a need for a maxillo-facial unit, and one was set up for him in the British Hospital at Wimereux. However, he was only supposed to operate under the supervision of a qualified surgeon, but his work so impressed Gillies that he was moved to investigate the subject further.

It being, as Gillies observed, 'a rather informal war', he was able to get hold of a book on jaw and facial injuries by the German, Lindemann. Then, during a period of leave, he decided to visit Morestin at the Val de Grace Hospital in Paris, as it was rumoured that he was performing miracles of surgical reconstruction with skin flaps and cartilage grafts. Morestin, an unpredictable Creole, received him kindly, and as Gillies watched him operate, to use his own words, he 'fell in love with the work on the spot'.

By the end of 1915, it was decided that Captain Gillies should proceed to the Cambridge Military Hospital at Aldershot to set up a plastic surgery unit. Whilst waiting for his department to be equipped, he revisited Morestin, who declined to admit him to his department! This waiting period was put to good use, however, for with his own money, he bought £10 worth of luggage labels, which he had addressed to himself at Aldershot. These were entrusted to the War Office, with the suggestion that they should be attached to the wounded soldiers who were then to be sent to his unit.

After a few weeks, the labelled patients began to trickle back to Aldershot, and when the Battle of the Somme reached its heights, 2,000 casualties, in place of the 200 expected, arrived in the space of 10 days. This massive influx of ghastly jaw wounds called for close teamwork, and together with a dental surgeon, Kelsey Fry, the unit began to emulate the results which the German surgeons, aided by Esser, were already achieving. There were no sulphonamides or antibiotics in those times, nor were there many standard procedures to follow, for civilian wounds of these dimensions were virtually unheard of.

In 1917, the unit moved to the Queen's Hospital, Sidcup, in Kent, where Gillies had been largely responsible for planning the hospital so that wards radiated from a covered oval passageway, in whose centre were the operating rooms and dental, X-ray and administrative sections. Here, in the 600 beds available, teams of surgeons from Australia, New Zealand, Canada and, later, America came to observe, learn and treat their own wounded.

The volume of work was enormous, but Gillies' energy and ingenuity proved equal to the daunting task with which he was confronted. There was no choice but to adopt the famous advice which John Hunter had given Jenner: 'Why think? Why not carry out the experiment?' Early on, Gillies, who had originally tried to close facial defects by direct suture or local advancement flaps, realised that where a piece of the puzzle was missing, new tissue had to be imported from elsewhere. It soon became apparent to him too that the lining of cavities such as the nose and mouth was just as important as the outer covering. In all, more than 11,000 major operations had been performed by Gillies and his team by the end of hostilities, and this vast experience had revolutionised the nursing care, the dental and reconstructive surgery and the anaesthetic techniques of that era. This was a grim reminder of the Hippocratic dictum that 'War is the best school for surgeons'.

Whilst the unit was still located at Aldershot, Gillies discovered that Henry Tonks, a well-known artist and teacher at the Slade School of Fine Arts, was working in the orderly room. Tonks, a fellow of the Royal College of Surgeons, had turned to art after losing his taste for surgery, and he was soon persuaded by Gillies to become the unit's artist. His appointment was expeditiously arranged by Sir William Arbuthnot Lane, a surgeon with a weighty reputation, who was the consultant to whom Gillies was answerable. Tonks' pastels were the basis of the invaluable pictorial records from which Gillies drew so freely to plan and illustrate his work as well as to teach the developing principles. Many of Tonks' drawings appeared in Gillies' first book, *Plastic Surgery of the Face,* and today, a collection of Tonks' original work is kept at the Royal College of Surgeons in London.

Not all the cases treated by Gillies in those days were gleaned from the French battlefields. In 1916, severely burned naval casualties from the Battle of Jutland were dispatched to him, and he also treated burns in members of the Royal Flying Corps.

This, then, was part of the foundation on which modern plastic surgery has been built, and in England, the men that Gillies attracted formed the nucleus of the specialty which has spread throughout the world along with the early work of continental surgeons such as Morestin, Lexer, Joseph and Esser to name but a few.

During the war years, much of the reconstructive work revolved around the tube pedicle, which has been rendered largely obsolete by the development of modern techniques. The idea was discovered independently by Filatov and Gillies at about the same time, although the Russian's publication in 1917 preceded the account of this innovation by Gillies, who later confessed to bitter disappointment when he learned that he had been beaten to the post. There can be little doubt, however, that Gillies deserved the acclaim he received for applying the technique so successfully on such a large scale and for spreading his knowledge throughout the world. It is hoped that he found some solace in the words of Sir Francis Darwin, who wrote, 'In science the credit belongs to the man who convinces the world, not to the man to whom the idea first occurs'.

In 1919, Kilner, who had proved himself a very capable surgeon in charge of a unit specialising in fractured femurs, joined Gillies at Sidcup and so began a close and fruitful association that was to last for the next ten years. Gradually, the wards began to empty, and in place of the soldiers, a few civilians appeared. Gillies' appointment with the R.A.M.C. ended in 1919, but he and Kilner continued to treat patients at Sidcup until the remaining cases were moved to Queen Mary's Hospital, Roehampton.

Between the Wars

It was a bold decision to decline his old chief Rees' offer to rejoin him in private practice once the war ended, but he had resolved to fully commit himself to plastic surgery, and instead, he accepted a somewhat lowly post at Barts, where Harmer referred cases needing plastic surgery to him. A private consulting room was rented in Portland Place, where, with Kilner as his assistant, the hard struggle began under precarious circumstances. In 1921, an article in *The Lancet* doubted if there was a place for plastic surgery in a general hospital, but by degrees, things began to improve, in some parts due to the motoring boom and its attendant accidents.

Birth deformities and burns, as well as nose and breast corrections, began to come his way. Although he held honorary appointments at the Prince of Wales Hospital and St. Andrew's Hospital, Dollis Hill, private practice was his only means of support. In 1923, the *British Medical Journal* announced that a fund of £25,000 was to be raised to build a plastic surgery wing at St. Andrew, and this was the first hospital in London to provide free places for plastic surgery patients. It seemed that Gillies' struggle to achieve recognition for his specialty was at last being rewarded, despite the fact that some spoke of him as a charlatan!

New rooms were found at 56 Queen Anne Street, in a splendid Adam house complete with a rather pompous butler named Peel. Gillies still had enough time upon his hands to practise golf in the waiting room, where he wore a hole in the carpet! His secretary, Robert Seymour, who had been patched up by Gillies during the war, took charge of the financial matters as Gillies had little money sense, although the practice began to become increasingly healthy during the late 1920s. Many patients were sent by dentists; the fee for a 10 minutes consultation was 2 guineas, and an operation could bring as much as 150 guineas. By the end of the 1930s, when his powers were perhaps at their zenith, he was said to be earning as much as £30,000 per year.

Besides his practice, Gillies was busy writing papers for *The Lancet* and *The British Medical Journal*, addressing medical societies and serving in an honorary capacity at several hospitals in and outside London. At last in 1930, he was appointed as Consultant Plastic Surgeon to his old hospital, St. Bartholomew's, and was generously granted two beds! Slowly, teaching hospitals throughout the country followed suit until, at the time of his death, there was scarcely one without its own plastic surgeon.

In 1931, to the delight of most of his friends and colleagues, he was knighted. Although he had been awarded the C.B.E. in 1920, it was thought by many that he was long due for some higher honour. His brilliant ideas, meticulous and dedicated work as well as his warmth and generosity had secured his position as one of London's busiest surgeons. Gillies would frequently refuse or return fees to those whom he considered needy, and despite his eccentricities, he was universally worshipped by his patients.

In 1931, Archibald McIndoe arrived in England from the Mayo Clinic. At this time, Kilner having set up by himself on the third floor of the London Clinic, Gillies was in need of a new assistant. In a sense, the loss of Kilner for Gillies was plastic surgery's gain in the form of McIndoe. Initially, Gillies helped McIndoe find a hospital appointment and subsequently took him on as his assistant. McIndoe believed that Gillies was a distant cousin, but Gillies was not sure and remarked, 'If so, very distant!' It was about this time that Rainsford Mowlem, also a New Zealander, fell under the spell of plastic surgery, and he along with McIndoe were ultimately taken into partnership by Gillies. This association lasted until the outbreak of the Second World War and was dissolved thereafter.

One further member of the team worthy of mention was the anaesthetist, Ivan Magill, who had joined Gillies at Sidcup in 1919. Although his first attempt to pass an endotrachael tube was abandoned after 1 hour, he later perfected the technique and developed a style and standard of safe anaesthesia that can truly be said to have served as a launching platform for today's sophisticated techniques. Magill conducted his work in an atmosphere of quiet efficiency, and on one occasion, he administered an anaesthetic in Paris, for a surgeon who was used to operating amidst a storm of froth, blood and coughing, since the anaesthetist was usually nothing more than a porter in possession of a bottle of chloroform. The intubation and the anaesthetic proceeded so smoothly under Magill that one of the French surgeons, who had never seen such a tranquil patient, was heard by Magill to whisper, 'Il ne respire plus. Il est mort'. Gillies and Magill were firm friends, but the former discouraged conversation with the anaesthetist, especially from visitors or assistants, and was known to reprimand his colleague if too much talking took place.

The Second World War

With the outbreak of the Second World War, Gillies, in his capacity as consultant adviser to the Ministry of Health, proposed that he and his three colleagues should train a series of maxillo-facial teams, and so was born the second generation of English plastic surgeons, men such as Battle, Barron, Champion, Clarkson, Oldfield, Heanly, Fitzgibbon and Hynes. Rooksdown House, part of the Park Prewitt Mental Hospital near Basingstoke, was chosen by Gillies as the location for his unit, where he and his team treated war victims from all the services as well as from the civilian population. Here, Gillies worked in an improvised operating theatre, which was partitioned off from a passageway.

Gillies had accepted responsibilities from the Ministry of Health, the Army and the Royal Navy and was given the rank of Honorary Brigadier in the R.A.M.C. McIndoe at East Grinstead concentrated on the treatment of rather glamorous burned fighter pilots, the famous Guinea Pigs, and his rising reputation began to eclipse that of Gillies, for the younger man's skill as a surgeon and organiser matched his burning ambition. Gillies' war work at Basingstoke was nonetheless admirable, and like McIndoe, he realised the importance of the social reintegration of his patients, and to this end, he helped establish the Rooksdown Club, which flourished under his patronage for many years after the war had ended.

The Surgeon

Gillies' style of surgery could probably best be called spectacular. There is no doubt that he was a good, if not masterly, technician, and if the need arose or the mood took him, he could be swift and decisive. But his unorthodox and innovatory make-up could involve him in tedious and time-consuming manoeuvres. His well-known habit of removing all the skin sutures at the end of some procedure in order to slightly rearrange the position of a flap is but one example. Kilner, on the other hand, had a set ritual for each operation, and his operations proceeded in regimented meticulousness with practised efficiency, which were characteristic of the man.

There is scarcely a subject in modern plastic surgery to which Gillies has not contributed something. Although it has been said by a cynic that 'the tube pedicle was his greatest disservice to modern plastic surgery', the idea still on rare occasions has its applications. He devised a number of flaps, including the fan flap, cocked hat flap for thumb reconstruction and variations on the forehead flap. His inlay graft for the correction of nasal deformities caused by leprosy produced spectacular results, but the same could be said of much of his reconstructive work. The views of modern society have vindicated his courageous and prophetic stand in favour of cosmetic surgery, and the nasal, abdominal and breast operations that were in the 1920s and 1930s so frowned upon are nowadays fully accepted. It was he who, in the face of opposition, strongly advocated breast reconstruction following amputation for cancer, but it has taken almost 50 years for the world to come round to his way of thinking. Innovations in cleft lip and palate surgery took their place in his repertoire, besides such daring procedures as osteotomies of the facial skeleton, which have only recently been taken up again and perfected by Tessier. His compassion drew him into the troubled waters of intersex surgery, and his patient attempts at penile reconstruction have only slowly been improved upon. But perhaps his most valuable contribution to surgery was in laying down and disseminating through his own energy the fundamental principles of his specialty.

Literary Inclinations

Gillies was not a great reader, not that there existed much in English on his subject to be read. There was a considerable volume of literature in French and German from Moresin and Esser, of which he was not at first aware. Apart from a few books, he favoured mostly medical journals; however, for the greater part of his life, there were no journals devoted to plastic surgery apart from the *Revue de Chirurgie Plastique* and the ill-fated *Plastica Chirurgica*. Prior to the establishment of the *British Journal of Plastic Surgery* in 1948 and its American equivalent, most of his publications appeared in *The British Medical Journal*, *The Lancet* or the *Proceedings of the Royal Society of Medicine*. He wrote two books: the first, *Plastic Surgery of the Face,* published in 1920, was largely based on his experiences in the Great War. A copy of this book, which was kept in the operating theatre at Rooksdown House, almost led to some unpleasant publicity for Gillies. The 'bible' went missing, and Gillies suspected that one of his assistants had stolen it. An intensive search proved fruitless, and Gillies injudiciously decided to break into the suspect's bedroom whilst he was absent from the hospital. The book was not there and in fact was later unearthed beneath a pile of papers and magazines in a coffee room, but the wronged party decided to proceed against Gillies for slander. The case was eventually settled out of court, Gillies agreeing to pay the young man £75.

His second book, *The Principles and Art of Plastic Surgery*, written with Ralph Millard, one of his old trainees, and begun in 1952, was published in 1957, and though Gillies was obliged to contribute towards the production expenses at the time, the book is still selling. In the late 1950s, although in some need of money, he turned down an offer of £6,500 by a Sunday newspaper to write a series of articles on his life. This was in conformity with the rigid ethical principles of the period, which have also robbed us of what would undoubtedly have been a valuable and diverting piece of history.

Teaching and Training

In 1939, there were only four fully qualified plastic surgeons in Great Britain, but many American surgeons had been initiated into the specialty of plastic surgery during the war years, and they and their colleagues continued to visit Gillies and his group in England during the 1920s and 1930s at St. Andrew's Hospital, Dollis Hill, and St. James's Hospital, Balham. His friends from America, Ferris Smith, Blair, Ivy, Risdon, Dorrance, Sheehan, Kanzanjian, Webster and Bunnel, read like a Who's Who in plastic surgery. It is thus obvious that most of his trainees in plastic surgery came from abroad, and perhaps this situation was in part encouraged by Gillies, Kilner, McIndoe and Mowlem, who subconsciously may have enjoyed their monopoly. They were prepared to travel widely within the country, sometimes to see and treat acute cases. For many years, Kilner, for example, spent three weekends out of four working in Manchester, Birmingham and Alton, whilst Gillies likewise operated and saw patients at Alton, Stoke-on-Trent, Birmingham and Leeds in the weekend.

Gillies preferred to hold the centre of the stage, whether it was in the operating room, wards or his own office, where his careful preoperative planning formed the basis of his own peculiar style of teaching. Not that he always adhered to these plans; for those who knew him less well, such capricious behaviour could be both puzzling and exasperating. His unique methods of instruction combined cajolery, invective, wit and raillery, but they left a deep and lasting impression on those who came to learn.

Amongst his many aphorisms which stamped themselves indelibly on the minds of his students were

- 'Never do today what can honourably be put off until tomorrow!'
- 'The great ignominy is that plastic surgeons cannot remove a scar without leaving another'.
- 'Never stand when you can sit down...'
- And, to a tiresome questioner, 'I never always do anything'.

The above and others constitute what Fitzgibbon listed as 'The Commandments of Gillies'.

Fame brought with it invitations to teach and operate in many countries, and for this purpose, he travelled widely in South America, Europe, Australia, America and India and such far-flung places as Nepal and New Zealand, where this author remembers a spellbinding lecture delivered at the Otago Medical School in 1955. His popularity as a lecturer was enhanced by his sense of humour and also by the free use of photographs. He was a pioneer in the field of clinical photography and was the first leading surgeon in the field of clinical photography and the first leading surgeon to encourage the use of the cine-camera in the operating theatre. Besides being the co-founder and President of the Medical Art Society, he became Chairman of the Medical Group of the Royal Photographic Society.

In 1944, Gillies conceived the idea of forming a British Association of Plastic Surgeons. The first meeting was held 2 years later, with 40 founder members and Gillies in the Chair. The association became affiliated to the Royal College of Surgeons of England, and in 1948, Gillies, together with Mowlem and McIndoe, contributed the first three articles to the *British Journal of Plastic Surgery*. On his 70th birthday, which marked his retirement from Rooksdown, the Association gave him a dinner, something he had vainly expected from the Garrick Club, and presented him with a silver George II tankard.

He was closely involved with the establishment of the American Association of Plastic Surgery, of which he was made an honorary fellow in 1934, and unhappily did not live to receive the Honorary Citation awarded to him by the American Society of Plastic and Reconstructive Surgery in 1960. In 1958, the *American Journal of Surgery* dedicated a commemorative issue to him, in which tributes from many of his old trainees and colleagues give an idea of the esteem in which he was held throughout the world.

The Artist

Of all his many talents, painting ranked not highest on the list. From his sketches, it is apparent that he was an indifferent draughtsman, and in his first oil painting, his children were unable to identify the animal which he intended to represent a donkey! Having dabbled in water colours, he turned to oils when confined to bed by an attack of phlebitis in 1933. Bernard Adams, whose fine portrait of Gillies fishing is well known, taught him the rudiments of the art, at which he became proficient enough to mount two one-man exhibitions at Foyles. At the second in 1959, 30 of his paintings were sold, and his work, mainly consisting of landscapes, is now highly prized and has found homes in many parts of the world, from Malmo to Miami.

The Inventor

As a lad, Gillies was a clever wood carver, and this ability to conceive and work in three dimensions was of undoubted use to him as a plastic surgeon. He was an inveterate inventor, and many of the surgical instruments which he designed, including his forceps, fascia stripper, skin hooks and osteotomes, are still in use today. The most ingenious of them all, however, is his combined needleholder-scissors.

Outside the world of surgery, his mind was constantly toying with the solution of varying problems. He designed a motorcar seat which swung out when the car door was opened but was disappointed to learn that many such ideas had been patented.

His aid-to-walking machine and electric razor improvement, although ingenious, were both deemed financially unattractive. One of Gillies' more successful inventions was the reverse coat hanger, which enabled the owner to hang his trousers above, instead of inside, his jacket, and sales of £1,700 were achieved at the Olympic Hardware Trades Fair in 1959.

The Sportsman

It is really not surprising that Gillies, who excelled in so many things, was also a brilliant all-round sportsman. His youthful preoccupation with cricket and rowing later gave way to golf and fishing, and he was a formidable, if infrequent, billiards player. During the 1920s, Gillies represented England three times against Scotland at golf, and in his heyday, he had a handicap of plus 2. In 1913, he won the coveted St. George's Grand Challenge Cup. Not only was he a superb player, but he was a golfing innovator, sometimes to the annoyance of the establishment. Long before the large-faced driver became popular, Gillies designed his own model with a 2 ½″ face, which he used to good effect. His notorious experiments with a high tee or the top of a beer bottle, offended the hierarchy at St. Andrews and gave rise to the cartoon which appeared in the *Daily Mail*.

Golf too was also an outlet for the most whimsical side of his nature. Gillies was not above substituting coloured balls or an egg for his partner's ball, and on one occasion, he bribed a greenkeeper to cut a tunnel from the hole to an adjacent bunker, much to the bewilderment of his opponents. One of his more outrageous practical jokes was perpetrated on the Royal and Ancient at St. Andrews, where he asked permission to play a round of golf in artificial light at night. Ostensibly, Gillies had been approached by the chief of the Aranaki tribe, which dwelt in an African forest in perpetual twilight, who was anxious for his people to learn the game of golf. Some 2,000 townsfolk, carrying Chinese lanterns, lit the course whilst Gillies and three friends played a round. He was later discovered helpless with mirth upon his back in the locker room at the thought of his ridiculous prank having fooled the prim committee! He played golf well into his seventies, but by degrees his handicap drifted into double figures, and he found it steadily more difficult to get around the golf course due to claudication.

As a fisherman, he confined his energies more to the serious side of the sport and to the enjoyment of nature. He was a member of the exclusive Houghton Club, which fished on what was said to be one of the finest stretches of water in England on the River Test in Hampshire. There, as nearly always in the country, he was accompanied by his black Labrador Retriever, and it was quite remarkable how often it was Gillies who carried off the honours after a day of fishing. Thanks to his assistants, he could find time to indulge his consuming passion for his favourite sports, and through them, he was able to relax and so return refreshed in mind and body to his work.

The Man

There must be few plastic surgeons unfamiliar with the bald pate of Gillies, below which the clear, brown, quizzical eyes look out above the half-lens glasses. A centurion's nose surmounted a grizzled moustache, and there was an odd pucker to his lower lip and chin, which seemed to presage a wicked smile. As a young man, he had dark brown hair, which, as it thinned, slowly turned grey. He was of above average height, with a head set deep between his shoulders, which accentuated the slight stoop he acquired with advancing years. His youthful slimness never left him even when he gave up smoking the 40–50 cigarettes per day, to which he had been accustomed for 48 years.

About town, he favoured dark, striped suits, which were discarded for tweeds or plus fours in the country or on the golf course. His legendary disguises took many forms, and knowing his love of practical jokes, one wonders if he kept an assortment of beards and costumes in his wardrobe!

Some of his pranks were quite delightful. When invited to lecture to the German Medical Society in Berlin in 1938, he had his speech recorded in German on three gramophone discs, which he arranged to be secretly played to the assembled toadies of Hitler's medical hierarchy, whilst he mimed the lecture on the stage. Each time a record was changed, he elaborately cleared his throat and drank from a glass of water. McIndoe was believed to have been hidden beneath a covered table at which Gilles stood. Sometimes at dinners, when his health was to be proposed, he contrived to secrete himself unnoticed beneath the table, to the confusion of his friends, whose search for him in the hall and cloakrooms proved fruitless. Jokes involving rolls of lavatory paper at the Garrick Club in the presence of royalty were not universally appreciated, and it was there that he demonstrated his ingenious coat hanger in 1951, much to the horror of the ladies, by removing his coat and trousers during a dinner party.

He took enthusiastically to motoring, which was invented in his lifetime, and was extremely fond of his Bentleys. When he lived in Hampstead, he often tried to coast his car to Regents' Park without the use of the motor, and success was achieved only at the cost of violating the traffic regulations.

It seemed that he delighted in breaking rules, and as a corollary, he was often exasperatingly late for operating sessions. Once begun, an operation proceeded with no regard for the time it took, until Gillies was perfectly satisfied that the best possible result had been achieved. It can hardly be said that his mischievous and unpredictable nature encompassed true laziness, for he continued to perform three to four operations a day and to travel abroad until the age of 78, the year of his death.

At the age of 75, he married his private theatre sister, Miss Marjorie Clayton, to many affectionately known as Sam. They were working together when his last illness overtook him, and he was admitted, following a stroke, to the London Clinic, where he so long had treated others. It was there he died, as the bells of the Marylebone Parish Church chimed half past seven, on the evening of 10 September 1960.

Of the many obituaries appearing in the British national press and medical journals on both sides of the Atlantic, none captures his charming and inventive spirit better or more eloquently than that of his old friend, Jerome Webster.

In 1961, an appeal was launched for a memorial fund, and a portrait of Sir Harold, which hangs in the Royal College of Surgeons, was commissioned. In the same year, the British Association of Plastic Surgeons decided to perpetuate his memory by the institution of a biennial Gillies' Memorial Lecture, together with the presentation of a gold medal. Kilner was the first recipient of this honour in 1961, and on each occasion, the lecture is published in the *British Journal of Plastic Surgery,* and although the rays are dimming, a little more light is shed upon the fascinating story which revolved around the 'Mastermind of Modern Plastic Surgery', Sir Harold Delf Gillies.

Chapter 16
Thomas Pomfret Kilner (1890–1964)

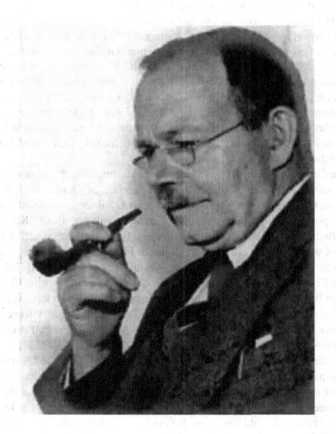

Thomas Pomfret Kilner was born on 17 September 1890, the son of a schoolmaster at Manchester Grammar School. He was educated at Queen Elizabeth's Grammar School in Blackburn, a busy cotton-weaving centre, which lies about twenty miles

© Springer International Publishing Switzerland 2015
D. Tolhurst, *Pioneers in Plastic Surgery*, DOI 10.1007/978-3-319-19539-1_16

to the north-east of Manchester. Besides its cotton trade and manufacturing industries, Manchester is well known for its university, and it was there that Kilner studied medicine, winning the Dauntesey Scholarship and the Sidney Renshaw Exhibition, as well as medals in anatomy and physiology on his way to qualifying in 1912, with distinctions in surgery and pathology.

Following 2 years as a demonstrator in anatomy at Manchester University, he became a house surgeon at Manchester Royal Infirmary, with the intention of taking up general practice in Blackburn. But the First World War intervened, and he joined the RAMC, first serving in a Casualty Clearing Station in 1915 and subsequently rising to the rank of Captain as a surgical specialist in No. 4 General Hospital. At the end of the war, he was placed in charge of a fractured femur unit, and having decided upon a surgical career, he was looking for a suitable job when his chief suggested there might be an appointment available in a new specialty: 'plastic surgery' with a Major Gillies at the Queen Mary's Hospital in Sidcup.

So in 1919 began the association that was to last for 10 years until Kilner struck out on his own. The story of Gillies' remarkable work is told elsewhere, but in Kilner, fate had provided him with an ideal partner, Gillies, the tall and elegant natural sportsman, light-hearted, unorthodox and artistic colonial was the antithesis of the short and portly, single-minded, hard-working and obdurate Mancunian. Both had brilliant minds, affected bristling moustaches and wore half lens spectacles, but there the likeness ended. Some said that had they stayed together, they could have conquered the world but in a sense, they did just that, for in England at least, there never was, nor has been, a partnership which so profoundly influenced the development of any branch of surgery.

With the Great War over, Gillies and Kilner continued the multistage reconstructive facial surgery on the victims of trench warfare at Queen Mary's Hospital, Roehampton. Gillies set up in private practice, with Kilner as assistant, and following a lean period, their unique work began to speak for itself. Kilner was an extremely dedicated worker and found little time for his hobbies, such as they were, but his chief was happy to escape the rigours of Harley Street, leaving his assistant to slave away whilst he relaxed with his golf clubs or fishing rod. At Sidcup, in the 'Garden of England', Kilner found time for beekeeping, but in the 1920s, plastic surgery kept him as busy as those objects of his erstwhile attention. Not only were the two busy in London, but they also travelled about the country to see and treat new patients and one weekend in each month visited Grocott to operate at Stoke-on-Trent.

Much to the disgust of Gillies, when Kilner decided to set up on his own in 1929, he took rooms two floors below Gillies at the London Clinic. It was not until the formation of the British Association of Plastic Surgeons in 1946 that they patched up their differences. However, in his second book, Gillies generously acknowledged the debt he owed to his old assistant. It was largely due to the close teamwork of Gillies and Kilner that plastic surgery in Britain gained a pre-eminent position in Europe and the British Empire.

Until the Second World War, Kilner worked at St. Andrew's Hospital, Dollis Hill, and it was not until the 1930s that the teaching hospitals began to show any interest in plastic surgery. He was appointed associate plastic surgeon at St. Thomas' Hospital in 1934, 2 years after Gillies had been allocated the princely total of two beds as plastic surgeon at St. Bartholomew's Hospital. Kilner continued to work and travel to the exclusion of nearly all else, visiting Birmingham, Manchester and Alton three weekends out of four and sporadically other parts of the country, as the need arose. His acquaintance with Wardill in Newcastle blossomed into a firm friendship, and they worked together to perfect the operation for repair of cleft palates, which Victor Veau had originally suggested. It was at the Lord Mayor Treloar Hospital in Alton that much of his outstanding cleft lip and palate surgery was undertaken, and he continued to visit the hospital until his appointment at Oxford. Also, he was Consultant to the Shadwell Hospital for Children, but this was bombed during the war, and Kilner's records were destroyed.

These peregrinations brought neither direct fees nor salary, as hospital appointments were then largely honorary, but the compensation was the enlargement of one's sphere of influence. Loyalties developed, resulting in a flow of private patients, so that by the end of the 1930s, Kilner was established in a comfortable house at Highgate, to and from which he was chauffeured in his Rolls-Royce. In private, his team comprised an assistant who received £300 per year, a nursing sister and his devoted secretary Miss Campbell who was Wardill's sister-in-law.

At the outbreak of the Second World War, Gillies' recommendations were implemented, and four plastic surgery centres were set up with Kilner being given charge of the pensioners at Roehampton. New hospitals were hurriedly constructed throughout the land, many of which still survive as the National Health Service's legacy from the wartime building boom. One of these hutted establishments at Stoke Mandeville was allotted 100 plastic surgery beds to accommodate the civilian victims of the London air raids, as well as injured servicemen, and Kilner was assigned to the unit.

Here, he worked in close cooperation with the dental surgeon, Greer Walker, and his chief assistant was Richard Battle, who subsequently succeeded him at St. Thomas' Hospital and Roehampton. Amongst his trainees were Osborne, Reidy, Lewis and Humby, inventor of the guarded skin graft knife.

Humby, the son of a well-known London dentist, studied medicine at Guy's Hospital, and it was there, whilst still a student, that the idea of the modification to the existing razor knife occurred to him. He was a good-looking young man, with perfect manners and much in demand by society hostesses. His glamorous reputation was enhanced by the minor acting roles he took to help pay his fees, and he was not in want of influential and lady friends.

In his enthusiasm for plastic surgery, he overlooked the need for proper qualifications and training in general surgery and, in so doing, jeopardised his career in England. Denis Browne recognised his ability but somehow disapproved of him, especially when he learned that Humby thought Kilner's cleft palate surgery superior to his own. On the other hand, Kilner was flattered when Humby made his views known and did much to help him.

Disillusioned with England, he went to the Far East where, being in possession of a pilot's licence, he became engaged in an airfreight enterprise, which dissolved in a scandal surrounding the theft of spare aeroplane parts from a neighbouring British base. His influential friends and his worsening pulmonary tuberculosis saved his skin but his partners landed in gaol. Humby drifted from the West Indies to Australia in search of a healthy climate and ended his days in Sydney, where he thrived as a plastic surgeon amidst not altogether undeserved antagonism from his Australian colleagues.

In 1944, Lord Nuffield endowed the first chair of plastic surgery in Great Britain at Oxford University with a sum of £80,000. It was rumoured that Eastman Sheehan, who was friendly with Lord and Lady Nuffield, would be offered the position. However, there was strong opposition from some quarters, one reason being that he had proffered his services to Franco during the Spanish Civil War. In the end, it was Kilner he appointed, once he had ascertained that Peet, the plastic surgeon already at Oxford, had no objections. Stoke Mandeville and the Churchill Hospital in Oxford together were utilised by Kilner as the teaching unit, with Reidy and Peet deputising for him in the respective hospitals. Calnan was appointed Senior Lecturer and was responsible for much of the scientific work, including the writing emanating from the unit, for Kilner was becoming tired after steadily overworking for more than 20 years. Kilner himself wrote relatively little. In all, he published less than thirty articles, several together with Gilles. The most valuable contributions were his papers on cleft lip and palate surgery and articles dealing with some technical aspects of skin grafting.

Glancing through the catalogues of surgical instruments nowadays, one comes across seven or eight instruments bearing Kilner's name. His skin hooks and the short, sharp, straight scissors (which seem to have drawn their description from the designer himself) are in common use, but Kilner's needle holders, which were never particularly elegant, are no longer popular. The suture frame designed by Kilner to fit the Dott gag, according to some of his old assistants, is an apparatus of mixed blessings, and the reverse nasal chisel, which he alone knew how to sharpen, was never a popular instrument, as it had a nasty tendency to avulse rather larger pieces of the nasal skeleton than was altogether desirable!

The university provided an atmosphere to his liking, and as a fellow of St. John's College, he mellowed, devoting much of his time to wise counselling and committee work, both for his college and the medical faculty. He was a founding member of the British Association of Plastic Surgeons, had a good deal to do with the writing of its constitution and served as President in 1948 and 1955. In 1946, he was awarded the CBE and, in 1952, was appointed honorary consultant in plastic surgery to the Army.

After his retirement from Oxford in 1957, it was decided that the plastic surgery chair was a luxury that could no longer be afforded. Kilner retained the title of Emeritus Professor and was appointed to the General Medical Council. During the appearance of seven plastic surgeons before this body in 1961 on a spurious charge of advertising, he courageously defended his colleagues, although knowing this action would not be popular with the Council. Following the 'acquittal' of the seven, he offered his resignation, which was refused, and shortly thereafter, he took his place on the Disciplinary Committee until ill health forced his subsequent retirement.

This incident illuminates the character of Kilner, who was a determined fighter, not afraid to speak out for what he considered to be right! One could imagine that he was rather forbidding, but he had a sense of fun and was especially fond of witty and amusing stories, which were carefully noted in a small diary. Yet he could be equally difficult and cruel, especially if circumstances disturbed his orderly routine.

From the moment he awoke, he expected everything to proceed according to a preordained plan. His coffee was poured so that when he arrived downstairs in the morning, it was just cool enough to drink. In the hospital, everything had to be meticulously worked out that, in contrast to Gillies' unit, one adhered to the prescribed ritual. Once he had found a good method of tackling a problem, he stuck to it, and there was never any talk of experiments on patients! His favourite dictum, 'God protect me from the surgeon who changes his plan in the middle of an operation', mirrored his philosophy.

Hard taskmaster though he may have been, his assistants knew where they stood and such was the quality of his mind and the precision of his work that his training, though based on his inherent conservatism, was second to none. His registrars and pupils were soon injected with his energy and enthusiasm, and his reputation attracted famous visitors from many parts of the globe.

He was at his happiest when operating, and some thought his pure technical skill put him in a class above Gillies. His short, strong, stumpy fingers proceeded relentlessly with their task, even whilst he taught or chatted with the anaesthetist. He was a quick, neat and efficient operator and especially good in the mouth, where he excelled at cleft lip and palate work. Children meant a great deal to him, and besides the surgical side, he took a strong interest in the analysis of speech and was on the council of the Central School of Speech Therapy and Dramatic Art.

If he had a failing, it was in his almost obsessive quest for perfection in the administration of his unit. He was unable to accept the usual untidiness of medical men and spent far too much time in checking patients' notes and records to satisfy himself that everything had been neatly and completely documented. Lengthy pedagogical diatribes on the responsibilities and failings of his assistants were far from endearing.

Little time was left for recreation, since he developed and printed all his own clinical photographs, and besides making a drawing in the theatre of every palate operation, he duplicated it later at home.

Although he abounded with energy, one could not have called him fit. He smoked heavily, often whilst washing his hands for an operation, and never had time for more than a few hurried sandwiches for lunch. In his forties, he was operated on for gallstones by Sir Stanford Cade and suffered a severe pulmonary embolus during the convalescence. A less serious complication was the development of a small cyst, where a towel clip had been inserted, and his views on this practice later were frequently made known!

Apart from 3 or 4 weeks at the seaside with his family in the summer, his principal diversion was Freemasonry, and most of his junior colleagues were obliged to listen to his 'lines' which naturally had to be word perfect!

Tragedy struck twice in Kilner's family: first, when his young wife died as the result of an abdominal catastrophe and, again, when his son, Hugh, who had qualified as a doctor, died at a relatively young age whilst on active service with the Royal Air Force. Kilner remarried in 1926 and his new wife bore him two more sons.

In his retirement, he remained in Oxford and was fond of gardening. He survived a dissecting aneurysm of the aorta which struck him down whilst he was picking apples, but he died 5 years later in the summer of 1964, aged 73.

Chapter 17
Gustavo Sanvenero-Rosselli (1897–1974)

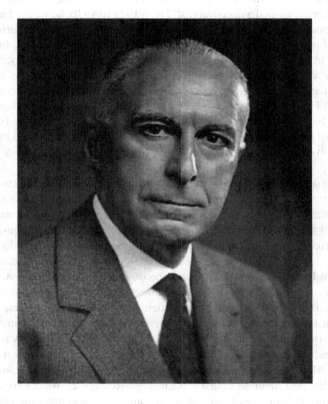

It is quite remarkable how many of the pioneers in the field of plastic surgery came from non-medical families. In this respect, Sanvenero-Rosselli was no exception for his father was a lawyer who followed the profession to which the family had inclined for several generations.

© Springer International Publishing Switzerland 2015

D. Tolhurst, *Pioneers in Plastic Surgery*, DOI 10.1007/978-3-319-19539-1_17

Sanvenero-Rosselli was born on 7 September 1897 in Savona, a busy port lying about 40 km to the west of Genoa, at the foot of the Ligurian Alps. It was there he grew up, the eldest of four children. He had two brothers, both of whom were to become lawyers in the family tradition, and one sister, who became the mother of one of Italy's present leading plastic surgeons. His father's untimely death left Sanvenero largely responsible for the family and life was far from easy. Although the income from government bonds was adequate at first, these were considerably devalued during the Great War, so that sacrifices had to be made when Sanvenero began his medical studies at the University of Genoa in 1915. His student days spanned the First World War, and for 3 years, up until 1918, he served as a medical orderly at the front. Despite this, he returned regularly to Genoa to take his exams so that he was able to complete his training within the prescribed period of 6 years and graduated in 1921.

During the War, he was thrown into contact with many cases of facial trauma, in which he soon developed a deep interest. From 1921 to 1926, he worked as an assistant to Professor Gavello in the ENT Department of the University of Turin. Gavello was himself involved in reconstructive surgery of the head and neck. In 1926, he was invited to lecture on this subject in a course in Madrid. Technically, Sanvenero was by now an ENT Surgeon, and although he had a brass plate made, he delayed putting it up and beginning a private practice, as his heart was not in a conventional ENT career. His mother and her other children were still somewhat dependent on Sanvenero, but he managed to shake himself free of the yoke of otitis (which was the subject of his first publication), ozena and tonsillitis and escaped to Paris where he had resolved to broaden his experience of the reconstructive work which he loved.

Besides a scholarship from Gavello's department, he was paid for lecturing in the ENT Department at the University of Paris, and thus he managed to make ends meet, whilst employed as a monitor in the ENT Clinic of Pierre Sebileau. The next step forward was the acquisition of a paid post as assistant to the bushy, black-bearded Fernand Lemaitre at the Clinique Internationale d'ORL et de Chirurgie Plastique de la Face. Lemaitre had been in charge of a large maxillofacial unit at Vichy where he had made the acquaintance of several allied surgeons, including Blair and Ivy from America. This acquaintance inspired him to invite the leading plastic surgeons of the time to lecture and demonstrate at a yearly course, which he organised in Paris from 1925 to 1928. Sanvenero-Rosselli availed himself of the opportunity to participate in the course in 1927 and 1928, and he was fortunate enough to meet such men as Victor Veau from Paris, Gillies from London and Ferris Smith, Ivy, Blair and Sheehan all from America, as well as Jacques Joseph from Berlin. During one of these courses, Sanvenero-Rosselli assisted Ferris Smith at several operations and, in general, made such an impression upon the latter that he made a gift of his surgical instruments to the young man. Sheehan too realised his worth and asked Sanvenero-Rosselli to accompany him on a scientific and medical tour of Spain in 1927. But in his turn, Sanvenero always acknowledged Ferris Smith and Sheehan as the two men who inspired him to turn from ENT to plastic surgery. Paris then was the turning point in his career, as it has been to countless others.

One morning in 1927, Sanvenero, as was his custom, opened the Corriere della Sera and, as he later maintained, was arrested by an article on the Padiglione per i Mutilati del Viso (The Clinic for Facial Disfigurements). This had been established by the City of Milan for the treatment of victims of the Great War with severe facial injuries, and because no one could be found to assume the responsibility of directing the clinic, it had regrettably remained empty. The heaven-sent opportunity was exactly what Sanvenero had been waiting for, and he returned to Italy and offered his services, which were readily accepted. In 1929, the clinic, comprising 25 beds and two operating tables which were housed in one room (as was for many years the practice at St. Bartholomew's Hospital in London), opened. Several months passed before Sanvenero saw any patients, but once they appeared, it was not long before the clinic established itself as Italy's leading centre for facial reconstructive surgery. Each year, at least two foreign residents spent a period training under Sanvenero, since such well-supervised posts were scarce in Europe, let alone Italy.

Besides the war injuries, Sanvenero began to attract congenital facial malformations, burned patients and facial tumours to the clinic. As the demands upon him increased, he began to visit outstanding specialists in the field of reconstructive surgery such as Lexer, Gillies, Joseph, Sheehan and Kazanjian in order to broaden his armamentarium. In 1933, he was appointed lecturer in the ENT Department at the University in Milan. There, he operated on the same sort of reconstructive problems which were related to ENT Surgery, such as tracheo-oesophageal fistulae and oral and nasal defects.

Following the establishment of the European Society of Reconstructive Surgery by the Belgian Coelst in October 1936, its first congress was held in Brussels in October 1936, Sanvenero being a member of the committee, along with Gillies, Kilner, Coelst and Esser. The second congress was held in London, and the third, at which Sanvenero presided, was held in Milan in September 1938 but was abandoned in midweek due to the Munich Crisis. The Honorary President was Pierre Sabileau.

The congress differed from their usual modern counterparts in that besides the presentation of papers, operating sessions were organised with demonstrations being given by such experts as Kilner, McIndoe and Sanvenero himself.

Under the gathering war clouds in the late 1930s, the Padiglione per i Mutilati del Viso was firmly established, and to mark its tenth anniversary in 1939, King Vittorio Emanuele III paid the clinic an official visit. Once Italy entered the War, Sanvenero devoted much of his time to the wounded, and in 1941, he organised the Centro Mutilati in Milan which was sponsored by the Sovereign Military Order of Malta and by the Italian Armed Forces. The centre was intended for reconstructive surgery to be performed on severe facial injuries in soldiers sent back from the front. In 1943, the centre was badly damaged by an allied bombing attack, and it was relocated in Lecco, on the eastern arm of Lake Como. Each day, Sanvenero and his theatre nurse went by train or drove the 40 odd kilometres from Milan to visit and treat patients, but the two were frequently obliged to walk or bicycle many miles due to closure of the road or interruption of the train service. On occasions, a car was loaned to Sanvenero by the occupying Germans who had commandeered the Villa d'Este for their headquarters in Northern Italy.

One can compare his work at this period to that performed by Gillies in the First World War, although Sanvenero had the advantage of being able to draw on a vastly increased store of knowledge. Nevertheless, his ingenuity and industry enabled many hundreds of facially mutilated soldiers to face life again with renewed confidence.

In 1944, Sanvenero received the shocking news that his sister and her husband had been killed in a car accident in Bolgheri, Tuscany. Their 6-month-old son Riccardo Mazzola survived. Sanvenero went to Bolgheri and collected the little child and took him back to Milan where he looked after him. Sanvenero's sister had joined the Red Cross at the beginning of the War, and besides working in Italy, she served in Albania and Russia. From this moment on, Sanvenero took a strong aversion to motorcars, and he himself never drove again, preferring to travel by train or taxi or to hire a car with a chauffeur.

The War over, Sanvenero immersed himself in the day-to-day activities of the Padiglione Mutilati in Milan, where he began to take a special interest in congenital facial deformities. Cases were sent to him from all over Italy, and his mounting experience and expertise soon made his name a byword in the field of plastic surgery. He accumulated a very extensive range of unusual deformities, which were carefully documented and photographed and now form the basis of the collection of his nephew, Riccardo Mazzola, who himself has developed a great interest in the same problem.

The magnitude of Sanvenero's experience can be gauged to some extent when one realises that he treated up to 180 new cases of cleft lip and palate per year. From this store of knowledge, he drew liberally both in the papers he presented at international meetings and in the 100 odd articles which he published, most of these being understandably written in Italian.

His first book, *Chirurgia Plastica del Naso*, appeared in 1931, and in the same year, he published an account of the activities at the Padiglione in the inaugural issue of Revue de Chirurgie Plastique. Sanvenero was a member of the editorial board of this journal, an appointment which he turned to good advantage when he founded the ill-fated *Plastica Chirurgica Journal*. This was designed to be the European sounding board of the specialty, and authors were permitted to publish papers in their native language, but after only three issues, the building housing and the printing plant were bombed, and the entire machinery was destroyed.

Sanvenero wrote quite a large number of papers connected with the specialty of ENT, which in the 1920s and 1930s was closely allied with plastic surgery. Cleft lip and palate surgery, tumour surgery, facial palsy and reconstruction following burns were subjects to which he made useful contributions, but perhaps his most valuable innovation was the superiorly based pharyngeal flap which is still very popular for the treatment of nasal escape in cases of cleft palate. It is described in his second book *La Divisione Congenita del Labbro e del Palato* (1934).

Sanvenero was a wise and patient teacher, and his appointments as lecturer in plastic surgery at the Universities of Turin and Milan in 1953 and 1955 were forerunners of the true recognition of his academic contributions. In 1962, the first chair of plastic surgery in Italy was created for him at the University of Turin, and in the following year, he was rewarded with a similar appointment in Milan. He was a member of nearly all the national societies of plastic surgery in the world, regularly attending and speaking at their meetings, and in 1967, he was President of the Fourth International Congress of Plastic Surgery, which was held in Rome.

To become an assistant of Sanvenero meant signing away one's right to a normal social life. The Chief regarded normal leisure hours as a heaven-sent opportunity to fit in more work or at least to study and woe betide those who failed to convince him that they shared similar sentiments. The normal working day began with the operating sessions at 7 a.m., and Sanvenero worked straight through until 7 p.m. when he went to his apartment for dinner. After the meal, he returned to the hospital and usually photographed patients until 11 p.m. He expected his assistants to attend these photographic sessions, much to their annoyance.

On Saturdays, he operated in private, but the wretched assistants were required to be present until he finished at around 2 p.m. On Sundays, he began a ward round at 10 a.m. and photographed outpatients again until about 3:30 p.m. At that point, he left the hospital saying to the team 'A good Sunday everybody'. Many patients believed that Sanvenero's instructions to attend the hospital on a Sunday were the result of an error, but to avoid confusion, he added as a footnote to his letter 'I will be present even on Sundays'. Sanvenero himself was in the habit of sending for far too many patients and frequently blamed his secretary, but she always smilingly showed Sanvenero the letters signed by him!

Although a bachelor, Sanvenero was particularly fond of children, and apart from his routine visits to the wards, he was often to be seen reading to and playing with his small patients. He had a knack of snapping professional shots of the children whilst conducting a sympathetic discussion with the worried parents. Sanvenero took all his own photographs not only because this was his main hobby but also because he was convinced no one could do it better.

In the operating room, he was a skilful technician and preferred to work in silence although he was prepared to answer questions posed by visitors. As a rule at least, four assistants scrubbed to assist him in the hopes of putting in one or two stitches or at least cutting a few, but even in this, they were frequently frustrated, as Sanvenero used a Gillies needle holder! His dynamic enthusiasm was particularly evident in discussion, and he remained receptive to new ideas throughout his long career.

After his retirement from the Padiglione (which changed its name to the Institute of Plastic Surgery at the University of Milan) at the age of 75, he continued to work in private practice and often treated free of charge those who could not afford his fees.

Work was his first love and he tended to regard holidays as a waste of time. He had no need of relaxation, but once a year, he took to the mountains where he climbed and walked right up until the year before his death. He always went to Solda in the South Tyrol and reserved the same room in the same hotel. This period was regarded as a working holiday, for he took the precaution of filling the station wagon, which he hired, with books and papers as well as his Olivetti portable typewriter. On occasions when his nephew accompanied him, there was scarcely any room for him, let alone his luggage!

Besides photography, Sanvenero was very fond of old books. Over the course of many years, he accumulated a priceless collection of rare medical books, many of which can now be seen at the Fondazione Sanvenero-Rosselli. The first edition of Tagliacozzi's book was acquired with almost his last penny in the early 1930s. He dared not tell his family what he had paid for it as the price was the same as that of an apartment.

Sanvenero was of medium height and slim build and looked rather drowned in his white hospital coats. His dark hair thinned at the temples, as it greyed, exposing a noble forehead, beneath which was a long face, strengthened by a bold nose. A sympathetic smile flickered frequently on his lips and his dark eyes radiated warmth and enthusiasm. Those who knew him well were struck by his aristocratic and cultured air which was born of wide travel and his appreciation of the arts. He was an intellectual who read deeply in the classics, such as Dante, Cicero and Leonardo. Besides a very formal type of Italian, sprinkled with quotations, he spoke fluent French as well as passable German and English.

A modest collection of Greek vases and antique furniture, mainly from Genoa, graced his apartment, where he seldom entertained. He preferred to go out to dine and was always in his box for the premiere at La Scala. Although he said he had no time for marriage, he was very popular with women of high society and went quite happily to their fashionable dinner parties. Good food, which abounds in Milan, was something he did enjoy. His wardrobe was extensive, and he had a large collection of suits and shoes and more than 700 neckties!

In his 75th year, he was as sprightly and as busy as ever, planning an issue for Clinics in Plastic Surgery. In the following year, he was to have given a series of lectures in New York at the invitation of Converse and Rogers. However, he died of pneumonia and complications, following an operation for a cerebral tumour on 17 March 1974, at the age of 77.

His nephew Riccardo Mazzola, who has followed in his footsteps, was largely responsible for the establishment of the Fondazione Sanvenero-Rosselli per la Chirurgia Plastica in Milan to perpetuate his memory. Most of Sanvenero's beautiful books can be found in its elegant library, which also has a fine collection of modern works on plastic surgery, as well as all the appropriate journals.

The Fondazione's aim is to foster the development of plastic surgery through meetings and lectures, which were regularly held at the magnificent Palazzo Visconti which no longer exists. Today, the Fondazione still organises well-attended courses that include live surgery, some of which are conducted in various hospitals in the city of Milan where Sanvenero-Rosselli spent the major part of his busy working life.

Chapter 18
Sir Archibald Hector McIndoe (1900–1960)

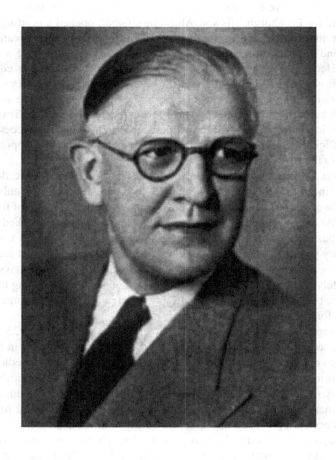

© Springer International Publishing Switzerland 2015   93
D. Tolhurst, *Pioneers in Plastic Surgery*, DOI 10.1007/978-3-319-19539-1_18

It frequently surprises me when the subject of plastic surgery is brought up that even though McIndoe died 55 years ago, the name of Archie McIndoe is nearly always mentioned. Many people seem to be living with the misconception that he was the founder of modern plastic or cosmetic surgery, if not in Britain then in the world! There is no doubt that he was a very successful and talented plastic surgeon with a forceful yet charming personality, but he was not the founder of the specialty. In fact in 1919, when McIndoe had just begun to study medicine in New Zealand, Harold Gillies had asked Thomas Kilner to join him as a partner in his plastic surgery practice in London. As explained elsewhere, it was unquestionably Gillies to whom the title of 'founder' belonged in Britain. During the First World War when McIndoe was still at school, Gillies became fascinated with the work of the Frenchman Morestin and decided to take up reconstructive surgery both during and after the war.

McIndoe's grandfather emigrated from Scotland and settled in the South Island of New Zealand where he took up farming on land close to Dunedin, the ancient Gaelic name for Edinburgh. His son, McIndoe's father, opened a printing business in Dunedin and married a strong-willed woman, Mabel Hill, who became one of New Zealand's most respected artists. She bore him three sons and a daughter, Archibald Hector being the second son. Archie, as he was called, was educated at the Otago Boys' High School, where in his last year, he became head prefect, sergeant major of the cadet corps and a member of the rugby and cricket teams. In later life, he took very little interest in sport and during the Second World War declined a commission in the Royal Air Force, to which decision he owed his success in side-stepping officialdom, red tape and bureaucracy when later he was appointed as a consultant to the Royal Air Force.

There was no medical tradition in the family, but in 1919, Archie decided to study medicine at the Otago Medical School which until 1965 was the only medical school in the country. The medical students were considered the elite of the student corps, and Archie was fond of parties and pranks but apparently worked just hard enough to pass the exams comfortably. It was at a party that he first saw a dark-haired, pretty young woman, Adonia Aitkin. She was a talented pianist and according to her it was love at first sight. They spent the rest of their student days together and ultimately married. Archie was an above average student according to his contemporaries, but during his final year, he showed signs of things to come when he won prizes for clinical medicine and surgery.

After completing the 5-year medical course, Archie qualified in 1923 and spent his 1st year as a house surgeon in Hamilton at the Waikato Hospital in the North Island. It was during this period that he received a letter from his old medical school informing him that he had been selected as a candidate for a scholarship at the famous Mayo Clinic in America. There are conflicting accounts about the exact train of events that followed. McIndoe later maintained that he was at first passed over, but after hearing the bad news, he was sitting with his head in his hands when William Mayo noticed him as he was walking through the university grounds. He paused and asked if there was something wrong, and when McIndoe told him how he had set his heart on going to the Mayo Clinic and how disappointed he was, Mayo was so impressed that he said 'I'll see what can be done'. On his way to

Dunedin, Archie had met Adonia, his sweetheart from student days in Christchurch, and they decided to marry on the spot. In due course, he learnt that Mayo had arranged a fellowship for him, but the terms of the fellowship stated that the candidates should be unmarried. McIndoe was thus obliged to leave his young bride behind, with the understanding that she would follow him whenever this could be arranged.

He began work as an assistant in Pathological Anatomy at the Mayo Clinic, in Rochester, Minnesota, on 1 January 1925 and published several papers on hepatic disease and biliary problems during the ensuing 2 years. After about a year, a position as lab assistant was arranged for Adonia who was able to join her husband. Once his surgical training began in earnest, he fell under the spell of Balfour, a Canadian who had been invited to join the staff of the clinic. Balfour's hobby was playing the organ, and when he discovered that McIndoe's wife, a talented pianist, had arrived, he was able to arrange a job for her in the Palm Court Orchestra of the Mayo Foundation's own hotel.

The family income of 45 dollars per week was now more than doubled, and with his promotion to First Assistant in Surgery, he seemed assured of a comfortable career in Rochester. Although he had profited from working with Judd and Balfour, both very experienced and fine surgeons, he realised that he would always have to play second fiddle to them. A short study trip to England and France as the J. William White scholar did nothing to change his plans for the future at the Mayo Clinic.

In 1930, Lord Moynihan, then President of the Royal College of Surgeons of England, arrived at the Mayo during a visit to America. Moynihan had been watching a brilliant young surgeon by the name of Adson remove a spinal tumour; however, he was more impressed with McIndoe when he saw him operating. Incidentally, the forceps designed by Adson were later to become popularised by McIndoe as part of the plastic surgeons' armamentarium. Later Moynihan suggested that McIndoe should come to London where there were plans to establish a new chair in general surgery at the Post-graduate Medical School and that this would suit him admirably.

Moynihan was a legendary figure in his own lifetime (as McIndoe himself was to become). An incomparable surgeon and teacher, he was a great showman and possessed a shrewd sense for making money. For example, one story tells of how he postponed a holiday to remove a wealthy woman's gallbladder on the condition that she paid him a guinea for every gallstone he found. He was fortunate enough to get over 900 stones and guineas out of her!

The persuasive tongue of Lord Moynihan appears to have hypnotised McIndoe who, lured by the promise of fame and fortune in London, later resigned from the Mayo and, now aged 31, departed for England in the winter of 1931. In England, all was disappointment; there was no new hospital nor Chair of Surgery, and Moynihan had only advice to offer. There was nothing for it but to begin studying for the fellowship examination of the Royal College of Surgeons since this qualification was a prerequisite for those aspiring to a surgical appointment in English hospitals.

At this time, Sir Harold Gillies, also a New Zealander, whom McIndoe believed to be a distant cousin (very distant according to Gillies), was in practice as a plastic surgeon in London, and McIndoe sought his help. Gillies was then instrumental in his being appointed as a lecturer in general surgery at the Hospital for Tropical Diseases. Sometime later after he had obtained his fellowship and continued as a general surgeon, Gillies offered him a job, first as an assistant in his practice, and later McIndoe joined him as a partner.

Once his interest had centred on plastic surgery, he resigned his post at the Hospital for Tropical Diseases in 1939. He soon held appointments as a plastic surgeon to St. Bartholomew's Hospital, the Chelsea Hospital for Women, the St. Andrew's Hospital and the Hampstead Children's Hospital. In addition to his private practice, he was also the consulting plastic surgeon to the Croydon General Hospital and the Royal North Stafford Infirmary and had been appointed Consultant in Plastic Surgery to the Royal Air Force. With such a string of appointments and considering the fact that there were then only four men specialising in plastic surgery in England, McIndoe was now firmly established. When war broke out in 1939, Gillies saw to it that four major centres were established in England. He himself chose Basingstoke, Kilner Roehampton, Mowlem St. Albans and McIndoe East Grinstead. Of the four, McIndoe was to become the most widely known due largely to his work with the severely burned airmen during the Second World War. To some extent, he also owed his fame to his gregarious nature for he was popular amongst members of the nobility, rich businessmen and actors. Even today, his name remains all but a household word.

It was now that McIndoe saw a chance to expand the recently rebuilt Queen Victoria Hospital, which soon began to shoulder the burden of treatment for the severely burned airmen who descended upon McIndoe from all over England. Although he had published papers on the operative treatment of congenital absence of the vagina and hypospadias, it was his work on burns that made his name. He condemned the long-favoured tannic acid treatment and introduced saline baths as well as perfecting skin grafting.

Not only burned airmen but also members of the other armed forces and civilians were treated at East Grinstead, but only those who had received their wounds whilst flying became eligible for membership of the famed Guinea Pig Club. The Club was originally christened the Maxillonians, but this somewhat pretentious title was dropped in favour of the Guinea Pigs, which was McIndoe's affectionate name for his patients. His surgical skill was one thing, but equally important were his farsighted and revolutionary schemes to rehabilitate his often grotesquely disfigured patients. He encouraged people in the vicinity to accept the young men socially and won battles to return them to active duty and later to self-supporting civilian jobs. The most famous of his patients at this time was Richard Hilary who, in his book 'The Last Enemy', gives a vivid account of what he and others suffered and of the debt they owed to McIndoe and his team. 70 years after the Guinea Pig Club was formed, it was still going strong – its members gathering once a year from many parts of the world to perpetuate the memory of 'The Boss' as McIndoe was known to many of his patients.

Even in 1969, I was privileged to operate on one or two Guinea Pigs who needed removal of unstable areas of skin or minor tumours during my training at East Grinstead.

Once the War was over, McIndoe continued his work at East Grinstead, which became perhaps the world's most famous training centre for plastic surgery.

In addition, he returned to his private practice in London where he greatly enhanced his name in the field of cosmetic surgery. The titled, rich and famous flocked to his rooms in Harley Street for facelifts, nose and breast corrections. Fortune followed fame, and besides the traditional Rolls-Royce, he invested in land on the foothills of Mt. Kilimanjaro, which was turned into a thriving farm through the labours of his partner, Robin Johnston. Once a year, he sought refuge from the pressures of London's social and surgical life in Kenya, but he invariably operated whilst in Nairobi, together with a wartime colleague, Michael Wood, who was to achieve renown as a flying doctor.

McIndoe published more than 40 papers, and it must be remembered that before the establishment of the *British Journal of Plastic Surgery* and the *Journal of Reconstructive and Plastic Surgery*, most of his articles had been printed in such journals as *The Lancet*, the *British Medical Journal*, the *Proceeding of the Royal Society of Medicine* or *The American Journal of Surgery*. His most noteworthy literary contributions were his articles on vaginoplasty, burns and breast reduction. In addition, he published papers on hypospadias, cleft lip, facial fractures, skin grafting and lymphoedema. The McIndoe vaginoplasty is still widely used, but the technique he described for the treatment of hypospadias has, like so many operations for this deformity, fallen into disrepute. Besides various skin hooks and a nasal chisel, the instruments of his invention which are now most commonly used are his scissors and non-toothed dissecting forceps.

During the Second World War, he was honoured by several countries and was a recipient of the C.B.E. in 1944. Three years later, he was knighted so one could argue he had reached the acme of his career 24 years after graduating as a doctor.

The nucleus of McIndoe's team, apart from himself, comprised his permanent theatre nurse, Jill Mullins, and a skilful anaesthetist, John Hunter. Such was the degree of understanding between him and Jill Mullins that they essentially operated in silence, each instrument arriving unasked for, so that his operations were conducted with beautiful fluency and at remarkable speed. McIndoe's fingers were short and rather thick, a characteristic not altogether unknown amongst masterly technicians. But his touch was sure, his experience was vast, and his energy and enthusiasm seemed to know no bounds, all of which took him to the very top of his profession. As if this was not enough, he combined a warm and generous personality with a splendid penchant for organisation, and it is little wonder he was elected to the council of the Royal College of Surgeons of England, which August body voted him Vice-President in 1958. Two years later, shortly before the election, in which it seemed he would be chosen as President of the college, a fellow countryman, Sir Arthur Porritt, was to fill the role with great distinction.

McIndoe excelled as a fundraiser and, in large measure, was responsible for the successful appeals which raised money to rebuild the Royal College of Surgeons following the war. His charm and fame enabled him to move in high and well-to-do circles. Amongst others, the Marks family, of Marks and Spencer stores, were both generous in terms of money and friendship. The burn centre at East Grinstead was endowed through the magnanimity of Neville Blond and his wife Elaine Marks. There is no doubt that all this and dedication of McIndoe to his profession made inroads on his private and family life, for his first marriage ended in divorce. However, he did embark again upon the seas of matrimony and found great contentment in his second marriage.

In 1943, his colleague and fellow countryman, Rainsford Mowlem, operated on McIndoe for Dupuytren's contracture in his right hand, from which he made a satisfactory recovery. Sometime later he underwent a laparotomy for persistent abdominal pain, and a swab was left in his peritoneal cavity, which subsequently caused him more distress but was ultimately retrieved. In 1957, his gallbladder was removed and it was also clear that his heart was not altogether in order. He underwent an operation for a cataract in Spain in 1960 and suffered further heart trouble during that year. One evening, following a dinner party in London, he returned to his flat with Lord Evans, the Queen's physician, where they sat up late discussing plans for the future. He retired late to bed and died that night in his sleep aged 59.

Chapter 19
Rainsford Mowlem (1902–1986)

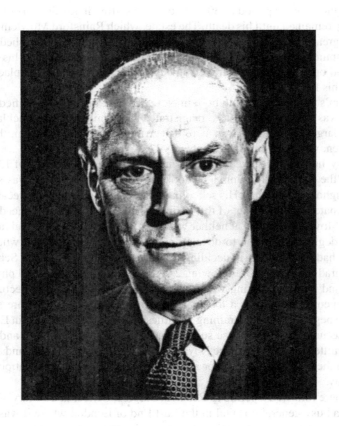

© Springer International Publishing Switzerland 2015
D. Tolhurst, *Pioneers in Plastic Surgery*, DOI 10.1007/978-3-319-19539-1_19

Rainsford Mowlem was the youngest of the four famous plastic surgeons who monopolised the practice of their speciality in England until the outbreak of the Second World War, and Mowlem, like Gillies and McIndoe, was born and grew up in New Zealand.

Mowlem's ancestry can be traced to one of William the Conqueror's soldiers, Durandos, who later took the name of de Moulhem. In return for keeping the King's tower at Corfe Castle in good order, de Moulhem received two and a half hides of land from the King, but in 1495 the land passed into other hands although the de Moulhem family remained in Swanage. By degrees, their name changed to the present form of Mowlem. When John Mowlem, Rainsford's great uncle, had made his fortune from contracting and demolishing business, he resolve to buy back the lost land which, by this time, was largely occupied by tenant farmers. A more agreeable landlord can scarcely be imagined for John Mowlem preferred to collect his rent in cheques which, over a period of 30 odd years, he stuffed in the drawers of a bureau, where they remained until his death. The estate, which Rainsford Mowlem inherited from his great uncle, was a sizable one and apart from the uncashed cheques included numerous bank accounts scattered around the world, which his eccentric relative had opened during his travels in case he ever returned to the places which had taken his fancy.

Mowlem's parents were both born in New Zealand; his father qualified as a barrister and was later appointed as a magistrate. The family lived in Auckland, New Zealand's largest city, and it was there that Arthur Rainsford Mowlem, the first of two children, was born on 21 December 1902.

As a boy, he was educated at a state primary school and, at the age of 13, became a pupil at the Auckland Grammar School, the reputation of which was second to none throughout the country. His schooldays passed lazily by in the agreeable South Pacific climate, giving no hint of the distinguished future which lay ahead.

Young Mowlem excelled at neither work nor games and his principal hobby was boats. By degrees, he began to develop an interest in medicine, and when he left school, he had no difficulty in deciding to study at the Otago Medical School from which he graduated in 1925. Following 2 years as a house surgeon and physician at the Auckland Hospital, during which time he made up his mind to become a surgeon, he spent 6 months as a locum tenens in general practice before sailing to England to begin his surgical training in earnest. Shortly after arriving in England in 1928, he secured a post as house surgeon at the Greenwich Hospital, and in 1929, he was admitted as a fellow of the Royal College of Surgeons of England. This was very much the classical formula for an aspiring specialist from the Antipodes, as it still is today.

Next, there followed a period as Resident Surgical Officer at St. Mary's Hospital, Stratford, a busy general hospital in the East End of London where it was possible to obtain a very extensive experience of general surgery in a relatively short time. This he did under the tutorship of men such as Milligan and Lawrence Abel.

At Christmas in 1931, Mowlem was on the point of returning to New Zealand when the Superintendent of the Hammersmith Hospital died, and a chance acquaintance, who knew Mowlem was free, asked if he would fill in for a week or two until a new man could be appointed. Weeks stretched into months, and opportunities loomed ahead which persuaded the young bachelor to postpone his return voyage.

Amongst his many honorary appointments at this time, Gillies numbered that of consulting plastic surgeon to the Hammersmith Hospital, and it was in a ward there that Mowlem first made his acquaintance. Quite understandably, until this time, Mowlem had jealously guarded the number of general surgery beds under his care against the incursions of the plastic surgeon. However, in a very short period of time, all this changed when he began to appreciate the work which Gillies was doing.

At the end of 1931, Gillies was offered the chance to establish a plastic surgery unit at St. James's Hospital, Balham with 25 beds, a dental laboratory, a secretary and ample operating time. Mowlem, who had become intrigued by the ingenuity of his fellow countryman's work, decided to throw in his lot with Gillies, and he moved to St. James's Hospital and was largely responsible for setting up what was to be the first real civilian plastic surgery unit in England. Besides Gillies, Kilner, McIndoe and Mowlem, there was a consultant dental surgeon and two consultant anaesthetists. Once the teething troubles were overcome, Mowlem decided to work part-time at the unit and accepted an offer to become Gillies' private assistant together with McIndoe. There was plenty of work, and Gillies' assistants soon had a fairly free rein in the practice, especially since Gillies was often away fishing or golfing!

As the new specialty of plastic surgery gained recognition, Mowlem, who had acquired honorary posts at St. Andrew's Hospital, Dollis Hill and Selly Oak Hospital in Birmingham, was appointed consultant in plastic surgery at the Middlesex Hospital in London in 1938, where, from time to time, Winston Churchill was admitted as a patient.

Then in 1939, the Second World War broke out, and Gillies advised the ministry to establish four new maxillofacial units. One of these, at St. Albans in Hertfordshire, was set up and organised by Mowlem, and there he carried on through the war years, treating both civilian and patients of the armed forces and training some of the second generation of plastic surgeons in England.

In 1953, the unit was moved to Mt. Vernon Hospital, Northwood, on the outskirts of London, not far from Harrow. Here it continued to thrive and develop under Mowlem and the brilliant team which he gathered around him. Then, as now, it attracted young surgeons from many countries, and it has maintained its name as one of the best centres of its kind in the world. Amongst the earliest of Mowlem's students were John Barron, Mansfield, Rouillard, Rank of Australia, Arneri from the then Jugoslavia and Honig from Holland. Later, Dawson, Harrison and Muir joined him, and when Mowlem retired, they consolidated the reputation Mt. Vernon Hospital had achieved under him.

After the war, most specialists worked part-time for the National Health Service and carried on a private practice. Mowlem's consulting rooms were at 149 Harley Street in the London Clinic where Gillies, Mcindoe and Kilner also had their practices. It was possible to earn considerable amounts of money in private practice as patients came to London not only from all over England but from many parts of the world. Mowlem worked closely with his own team, a secretary who fixed all the fees, a nurse and a steady stream of young trainees who, although employed by the National Health Service, were prepared to assist in private in their free time.

In 1933, Mowlem married Miss Margaret Harvey, and two daughters were born to the couple who established their London home in St. John's Wood. Later, Mowlem bought a country house in Great Missenden in the Chilterns. Such a lifestyle was possible through hard work and the steady stream of patients which his mounting reputation supplied.

Mowlem was not averse to cosmetic surgery, but he preferred reconstructive work, and although realising the importance of research, this only interested him if it had a direct bearing on surgery. His major scientific contributions were on bone grafting and the behaviour and formation of scar tissue and keloids.

The unit at Mt. Vernon Hospital was the meeting place for young and experienced plastic surgeons from all over the world. Teaching and travelling took second place to surgery which was his main interest, and he preferred to teach by example rather than by didactic methods.

At the age of 60, Mowlem decided to abandon his life and busy practice in England for the sun and peace of Spain. Both he and his wife longed for a warm climate, and his substantial inheritance meant that early retirement would bring no financial hardship. There was much speculation over the reason for his decision to retire somewhat earlier than is customary. Mowlem himself gave the answer when he said that the change between the war years, when everyone worked selflessly for the good of their fellows and the nation and the post-war period, which ushered in a gradual decline in integrity and idealism, was distasteful to him. He felt that there was too much self-seeking, jealousy and pecuniary interest in London and wanted no part of it. In the National Health Service, the decline in efficiency irritated him, and he had no wish to become a committee man as so many of his senior colleagues had and were doing.

By nature, Mowlem was a quiet man who was fond of reading and listening to music. When he moved to Spain, he developed an interest in gardening and irrigated his flower beds and orange trees by an ingenious but simple system of water works, which also filled his swimming pool from a spring in the hills above his house. He was also a good carpenter, and upon his retirement from Mr. Vernon, the staff presented him with a vast chest of carpenter's tools, upon which he commented: 'Not only are you retiring me, you're trying to bury me as well!'

Mowlem was of average height with brown eyes and dark brown hair, which thinned, leaving him bald in his forties. Although he dressed tidily, he was not interested in clothes. However, he did have a weakness for smart cars in his London days, owning Jaguars, Bentleys and an Aston Martin.

In 1959, it was decided that residual money from the International Plastic Surgery Congress should be invested to provide a travelling grant for young plastic surgeons. This was the Mowlem Award, and for many years, he maintained an interest in the development of his old profession and sat on the selection committee, but with the passage of time, he realised that his self-imposed exile made him unsuitable for such a task. In 1970, he relinquished this final connection with his old world and continued to live quietly and happily in the hills above Malaga in Spain, until his death in 1986.

Epilogue

Some readers may wonder what developments have already occurred or are taking place in the twenty-first century. However, it was our intention to write about the past and not the future. This century is still in its infancy, and so far there is little to add to progress made in the twentieth century.

It is not easy to make predictions of what progress will have been made by the end of this century. Even the experts in science and medicine do not know how nano-technology, bionics, organ transplant and tissue culture may be developed and applied to medicine, let alone to surgery. At present, for example, we are still occupied with improvements in microsurgery, such as joining together small blood vessels with a diameter of less than 1 mm. Tiny staples may be replaced by micro-sleeves or new glues, compatible with body tissues as they become available. Fibre optics and very small cameras are already in use providing possibilities for following results of various types of treatment and giving birth to new techniques. Special cameras are now even able to see through circulating blood.

When one realises that red blood cells are about 25,000 times smaller than grains of sand, it is virtually impossible to visualise such dimensions in comparison with what we can now see with the naked eye. The properties of new materials are still being revealed and their uses are yet to be applied.

Beyond these scientific revelations and applications, the imagination of the human mind seems to know no boundaries.

© Springer International Publishing Switzerland 2015
D. Tolhurst, *Pioneers in Plastic Surgery*, DOI 10.1007/978-3-319-19539-1

Index

Printed in the United States
By Bookmasters